The Body in Motion
Agility and Coordination

Fitness, Health & Nutrition was created by Rebus, Inc. and published by Time-Life Books.

REBUS, INC.

Publisher: RODNEY FRIEDMAN
Editorial Director: CHARLES L. MEE JR.

Editor: THOMAS DICKEY
Senior Editor: CARL LOWE
Senior Writer: BONNIE J. SLOTNICK
Text Editor: LINDA EPSTEIN
Associate Editors: MARY CROWLEY, WILLIAM DUNNETT
Chief of Research: CARNEY W. MIMMS III
Assistant Editor: PENELOPE CLARK
Copy Editor: ROBERT HERNANDEZ
Contributing Editor: JACQUELINE DAMIAN

Art Director: JUDITH HENRY
Associate Art Director: FRANCINE KASS
Designer: SARA BOWMAN
Still Life and Food Photographer: STEVEN MAYS
Exercise Photographer: ANDREW ECCLES
Photo Stylist: LEAH LOCOCO

Test Kitchen Director: GRACE YOUNG

Time-Life Books Inc. is a wholly owned subsidiary of

TIME INCORPORATED

Founder: HENRY R. LUCE 1898-1967

Editor-in-Chief: JASON MCMANUS
Chairman and Chief Executive Officer: J. RICHARD MUNRO
President and Chief Operating Officer: N.J. NICHOLAS JR.
Corporate Editor: RAY CAVE
Executive Vice President, Books: KELSO F. SUTTON
Vice President, Books: GEORGE ARTANDI

TIME-LIFE BOOKS INC.

Editor: GEORGE CONSTABLE

Executive Editor: ELLEN PHILLIPS
Director of Design: LOUIS KLEIN
Director of Editorial Resources: PHYLLIS K. WISE
Editorial Board: RUSSELL B. ADAMS JR., DALE M. BROWN, ROBERTA CONLAN, THOMAS H. FLAHERTY, LEE HASSIG, DONIA ANN STEELE, ROSALIND STUBENBERG, HENRY WOODHEAD
Director of Photography and Research: JOHN CONRAD WEISER
Assistant Director of Editorial Resources: ELISE RITTER GIBSON

President: CHRISTOPHER T. LINEN
Chief Operating Officer: JOHN M. FAHEY JR.
Senior Vice Presidents: ROBERT M. DESENA, JAMES L. MERCER, PAUL R. STEWART
Vice Presidents: STEPHEN L. BAIR, RALPH J. CUOMO, NEAL GOFF, STEPHEN L. GOLDSTEIN, JUANITA T. JAMES, HALLETT JOHNSON III, CAROL KAPLAN, SUSAN J. MARUYAMA, ROBERT H. SMITH, JOSEPH J. WARD
Director of Production Services: ROBERT J. PASSANTINO

FITNESS, HEALTH & NUTRITION

The Body in Motion

Agility and Coordination

TIME
LIFE
BOOKS

Time-Life Books, Alexandria, Virginia

CONSULTANTS FOR THIS BOOK

Ron Helman is a former competitive gymnast and coach who has also performed in mime and gymnastic dance. He has taught tumbling and acrobatics at the Juilliard School and is the owner and director of a studio of exercise and movement arts in New York City.

Richard C. Nelson, Ph.D., is Director of the Biomechanics Laboratory at Pennsylvania State University and a member of the editorial board of advisers for *Fitness, Health & Nutrition.* He is also an adviser on biomechanics to the International Olympic Committee and participates in studies of Olympic gymnasts.

Toby Towson is a six-time National Gymnastics floor exercise champion. An internationally accomplished teacher and performer of gymnastics, he is also the director of the Musawwir Gymnastic Dance Company and a contributing writer to *International Gymnast* magazine.

Nutritional Consultants

Ann Grandjean, Ed.D., is Associate Director of the Swanson Center for Nutrition, Omaha, Neb.; chief nutrition consultant to the U.S. Olympic Committee; and an instructor in the Sports Medicine Program, Orthopedic Surgery Department, University of Nebraska Medical Center.

Myron Winick, M.D., is the R.R. Williams Professor of Nutrition, Professor of Pediatrics, Director of the Institute of Human Nutrition, and Director of the Center for Nutrition, Genetics and Human Development at Columbia University College of Physicians and Surgeons. He has served on the Food and Nutrition Board of the National Academy of Sciences and is the author of many books, including *Your Personalized Health Profile.*

For information about any Time-Life book please call 1-800-621-7026, or write:
Reader Information
Time-Life Customer Service
P.O. Box C-32068
Richmond, Virginia 23261-2068

First printing.
Published simultaneously in Canada.
School and library distribution by Silver Burdett Company, Morristown, New Jersey.

TIME-LIFE is a trademark of Time Incorporated U.S.A.

Library of Congress Cataloging-in-Publication Data
The Body in motion.
    (Fitness, health & nutrition)
    Includes index.
    1. Exercise — Health aspects. 2. Fitness. 3. Gymnastics. 4. Motor ability. I. Time-Life Books. II. Series: Fitness, health and nutrition.
RA781.B63 1988   613.7   88-24845
ISBN 0-8094-6122-6
ISBN 0-8094-6123-4 (lib. bdg.)

This book is not intended as a substitute for the advice of a physician or an athletic coach. Readers who have or suspect they may have specific medical problems should consult a physician or certified physical therapist about any suggestions made in this book. As noted on page 21, certain exercises should not be performed without the assistance of a spotter.

CONTENTS

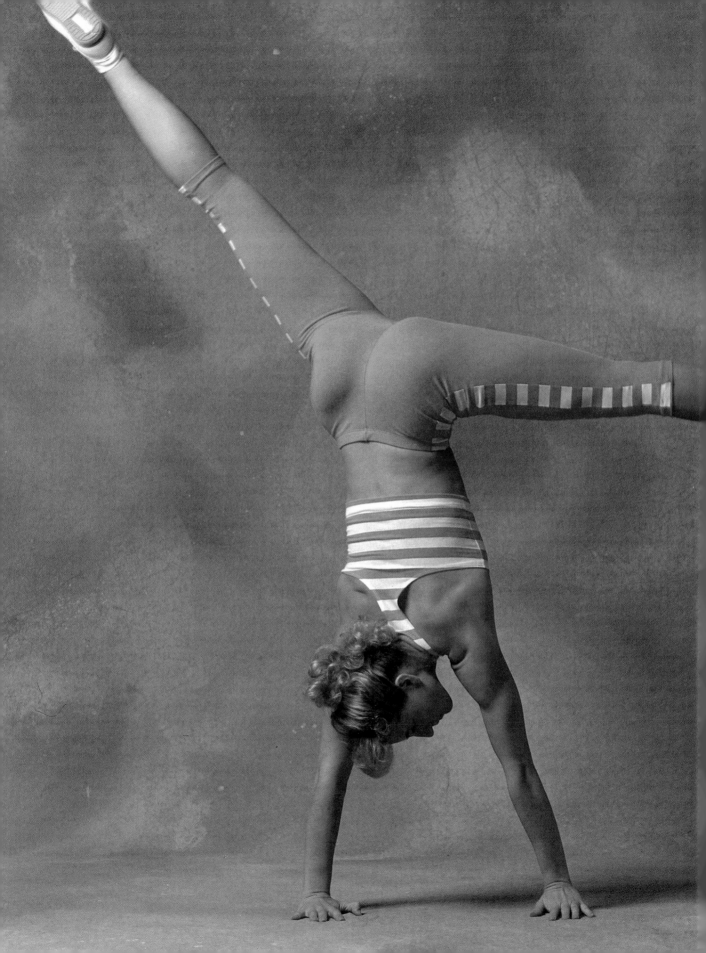

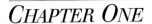

CHAPTER ONE

The Mechanics of Grace

*How your body learns and
masters movement*

Fitness is usually associated with strength and energy, and most fitness books concentrate on exercises aimed at building these two elements. However, every active person can also benefit from exercises that will enhance agility and coordination — two aspects of movement that are especially apparent when you exercise or engage in sports or other recreational activities. This book is intended to enhance your awareness of how your body moves, with exercises that will not only make your everyday motions more graceful, but that will also improve your athletic performance by making your movements more accurate and confident.

Even though much of the complex physiological activity necessary for movement proceeds unconsciously, all human movement requires a coordinated sequence of muscle contractions, changes in various joint positions and a variation in the tension applied to tendons and ligaments. Becoming aware of some of these movement characteristics is the first step to increasing agility.

Your Shifting Center of Gravity

The key to both motion and stability is knowing where your center of gravity is. Technically, this is the spot around which your weight is evenly distributed — your balance point.

In a sphere or a cube, the center of gravity is located in the geometric center. In an irregularly shaped object like the human body, the center of gravity is continually changing position as the body takes on new configurations.

When you stand erect (*right*), your center of gravity is located at a point just above half your height as measured from the floor. It is 1 to 2 percent higher in men than in women, since women usually have heavier pelvises and smaller upper bodies than men do.

As soon as you move, your center of gravity shifts by as much as several inches, as in the leaning and crouching figures (*far right*). For example, when you raise your arms over your head, your center of gravity rises two to three inches.

Sometimes your center of gravity is actually located outside your body: When you are curled into a U shape — the pike position in gymnastics — your center of gravity shifts to a point just outside and in front of your waist area, as in the diver (*center*).

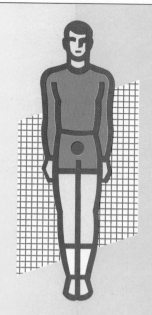

What makes you move?

You move when your nerves direct your muscles to contract: These impulses cause muscles to pull on the bones, to which they are attached by tendons, causing motion around the joint (or joints).

While much movement is the result of conscious effort, the details of that movement are determined by unconscious nerve and muscle activity. For example, you may consciously decide to raise your arm, but most of the pattern of muscle contraction and relaxation that actually causes the motion is directed by nerve impulses that travel from the peripheral nerves to the spine and then back to the muscles, as well as by brain impulses that do not engage your consciousness. This is quite practical: If you had to think about all your muscle activity, every movement would require so much thought and conscious control that you would have time to think of nothing else.

What distinguishes graceful from awkward movement?

The key characteristic of graceful movement is efficiency. Efficient motion is performed when there is no effort wasted on unnecessary muscular contractions or muscle tension.

For this reason, people who are just learning an athletic skill are often awkward; they attempt to control their motion too much, or in the wrong way, contracting an array of muscles that get in the way of graceful performance. For example, when a child learns to throw a ball, he keeps his arm muscles tight during the entire throwing cycle, thinking that the tension will ensure accuracy and distance. An experienced ballplayer, in contrast, initiates the throwing motion by contracting the appropriate muscles and then relaxing them for the

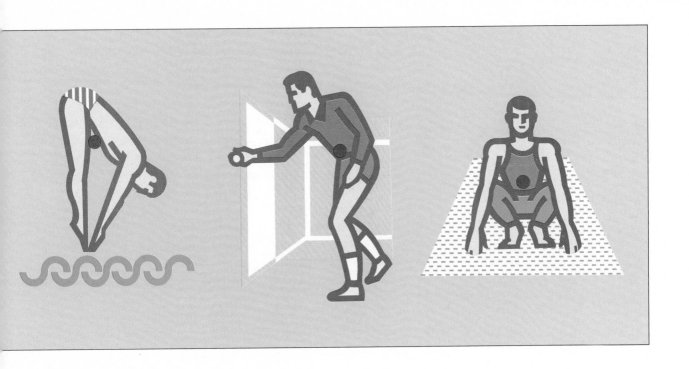

follow-through. The ballplayer's throwing motion is efficient, unlike the child's, and therefore, it is more graceful.

What is coordination?
When your muscles work together to perform actions in a harmonious way, your movement is well coordinated. While scientists who study human movement believe that much of a person's coordination potential is genetically determined, they also believe that experience has a great deal to do with how much of that potential is developed. The smooth interrelationship of muscles and nerves is the result of practice, as you can see clearly when you compare the awkward walk of toddlers, even those who will grow up to be very coordinated, with the graceful walking and running of a five-year-old whose movements are habitual and unconscious.

What is agility?
While almost everyone agrees that agile movements are actions that are well coordinated, efficient, quick, accurate and reflect confidence, researchers who have investigated human motion differ about how to assess and test this characteristic experimentally. Since agility also incorporates the idea of changing one's direction rapidly, one widely used test of this quality utilizes scattered markers through which subjects have to thread a path as quickly as possible. However, this test does not measure everyone's agility accurately, since agility can be very specific. It is possible to be an agile runner and awkward at sports that require jumping; conversely, proficiency at tumbling does not guarantee graceful skating.

Why is agility important?

Being agile reduces the effort necessary to perform movements. The excess contraction of muscles that impedes agility wastes energy. If you can avoid this unnecessary muscle use, you will find it easier to perform both aerobic exercise, such as running, and activity that relies on a high, short-term output of strength like weight lifting.

Improved agility can also enhance your performance in virtually all sports, especially those requiring rapid direction changes, like racquetball and tennis, and those that need a combination of complex physical skills, like basketball. When you are more agile, your timing and aim improve. You have more energy for performing the skills required by the action of the game when you do not waste it on the basic movements. For example, a beginning tennis player must use a great deal of energy simply trying to hit the ball, while an agile, experienced player has energy to spare for determining and carrying out strategy as the game proceeds.

In addition, when you perform athletic movements confidently and in a relatively relaxed state, your muscles, tendons and other parts of your body are less prone to stressful opposition from muscles that contract needlessly and impede your motion; thus, you are less vulnerable to injury. Unnecessary tension in the muscles opposing those you are using in your sport or exercise increases your chances of experiencing sudden muscle tears.

Is agility inherited or can it be learned?

No one knows exactly how much agility is inherited and how much can be learned. However, at least one study shows that even experienced, professional athletes can improve their agility through a rigorous training program involving movement. A study of the Dallas Cowboys professional football team showed that a conditioning program that emphasized movement skills helped many of the athletes become more adept at agility drills. When tested for how fast they maneuvered through a pylon course, these experienced players found that even after years of playing professional football, their agility still could be increased, and their times improved. You can only approach your inherent limits by frequent workouts and practice, as elite gymnasts do by exercising for many hours every day.

Learning agility means increasing your body awareness — acquiring knowledge about how your own body moves and reacts. While humans share some common characteristics in the way they move and react, every individual has his or her own unique traits. The more familiar you are with your physiological capabilities, the better you will be able to improve your agility and coordination.

What is body awareness?

Body awareness refers to your ability to judge accurately how your body positions itself or moves. Your proprioceptors — special receptors in your muscles, joints, ligaments, tendons and inner ears —

Keeping Your Balance

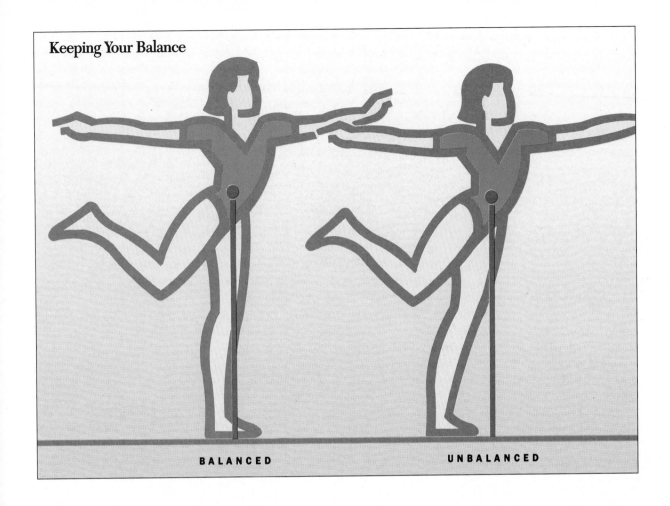

BALANCED   UNBALANCED

monitor the tension in your muscles, and the relative positions of your limbs, head and torso. Research shows that proprioception is a source of very accurate information about what your body does. For example, experimenters have found that you can differentiate between two disparate arm positions that are greater than 1.25 centimeters apart. Nevertheless, studies indicate that no matter how accurate your proprioceptors are, you still use your vision as your primary sensory information to tell you where your body is. This research demonstrates that even when your vision misjudges your body position and your proprioceptive information is actually correct, you still tend to obey what your eyes show you, overriding your proprioception in virtually every instance.

When you are balanced, your center of gravity is directly over your base of support; it is above or between your feet when you are in a vertical position *(above left)*. If you move and your center of gravity shifts too far in one direction or another *(above)*, you will lose your balance and have to move your legs to keep from falling.

What determines your sense of balance?

Your proprioceptors enable you to maintain your sense of balance, which is crucial to your ability to move quickly in any direction without falling. Experience has taught you the unconscious control of your muscles that keeps you upright while you move or stand.

A good sense of balance is vitally important for any sport in which swift, accurate movement is required. For instance, it is especially crucial in sports, such as ice hockey or basketball, in which you have to move and change direction at full speed while avoiding opponents, maneuvering a puck or ball. Maintaining your balance while you play without having consciously to think about doing so, enables you to revise your game strategy, concentrate on scoring or frustrating your opponents' offense.

What is the relationship between balance and center of gravity?
Your center of gravity is the point within your body around which all of your weight is evenly distributed. Since you constantly shift your arms, legs, torso and head, changing the distribution of your weight, your center of gravity is not in a fixed spot: It changes depending on your posture and position.

The location of your center of gravity affects your stability and equilibrium. You cannot be stable unless your center of gravity is positioned directly over the body parts that support you — feet, knees, hands or whatever. The higher your center of gravity is, the less stable you are and the more likely you are to fall. The lower your center of gravity, the easier it is to keep your balance. If you raise your arms, hold a weight on your head or wear high-heeled shoes, your center of gravity rises and you have more difficulty keeping your equilibrium. On the other hand, if you crouch down or merely bend your knees, your center of gravity drops, providing greater stability. Maintaining body stability and staying on your feet is most important during sports in which you are likely to collide with another body, but keeping your center of gravity as low as possible by maintaining proper body position is extremely important in all sports.

Performing tumbling exercises, such as those in Chapter Three, increases your sense of where your center of gravity is at different body positions and contributes to your ability to move quickly and change directions while keeping your balance. When you have a strong sense of your center of gravity over your feet, you minimize your chances of losing control of your movement and falling.

What is the quickest way to improve your agility?
Practice. The quickest, and, in fact, the only way to improve your agility is to practice the movements you wish to perfect, and to perform related exercises that work the muscles involved repetitively. While it also helps to have a good understanding of the muscles and bones needed for a particular movement, with practice, the muscle activity that enables you to be agile will occur below your level of conscious awareness eventually.

One of the most basic examples of this principle is evident as a child prepares to walk. He learns this movement not only by practicing actual walking but also by strengthening his leg muscles while crawling and rolling over in what are actually simple gymnastic activities. Although a young child does not understand the inner physiological functions of his muscles, he constantly observes the biomechanics of his body. His growing — albeit unconscious — awareness of his center of gravity results in the development of his sense of balance throughout his movement.

Similarly, when you wish to learn agility at a new skill as an adult, such as running, swimming or biking, you can do so by not only practicing the particular sport, but also by engaging in exercises like gymnastics that develop agility and work the same muscles as that sport requires. How fast your agility progresses will depend both on your perseverance at your regimen as well as your innate ability.

Gymnastic exercises that teach you how to stretch and reach in all directions make it easier for you to accomplish quick movements, no matter what sport you participate in, since flexible muscles offer less resistance to your movement. And even though much of your muscle quickness is genetically determined, the proper training can fine-tune your innate ability to react quickly and accurately.

How does your body learn to perform unfamiliar movements?
Scientists who have studied the movements of the human body believe that unfamiliar activities are under more of your conscious control than movements that you know well. For example, when you first learn to perform an unfamiliar motion, such as a gymnastic routine, you consciously direct that movement in response to feedback from your senses. Because you are unsure of yourself, you need to watch your body constantly, checking the position of your arms, legs and torso, to see that you are performing it correctly.

Some researchers think that over a period of time, after you practice and become proficient at a particular type of movement, a greater portion of your conscious muscle control switches gradually to the cerebellum, the part of the brain concerned especially with the coordination of muscles and the maintenance of equilibrium. Researchers believe this part of your brain, which operates without your conscious intervention, is better equipped to direct a familiar activity smoothly and accurately, with a minimal amount of correction.

After you have learned a complex sequence of movements, such as an intricate gymnastic or dance routine, some studies indicate that the simpler actions of your routine become automatic while the more difficult movements still demand conscious attention. Similarly, while performing an activity that demands responses to outside stimuli, such as hitting a baseball or driving a car, movements that follow a predictable pattern may proceed at an unconscious level. At the same time, sudden changes in your situation, such as being thrown a ball that curves in an unusual way, engage your attention at both a conscious and unconscious level.

What is the best way to learn a new movement?
It depends on how easily you can isolate the components of the movement. Learning how to shoot a basketball, for example, is best done by practicing the entire motion. The individual steps of that

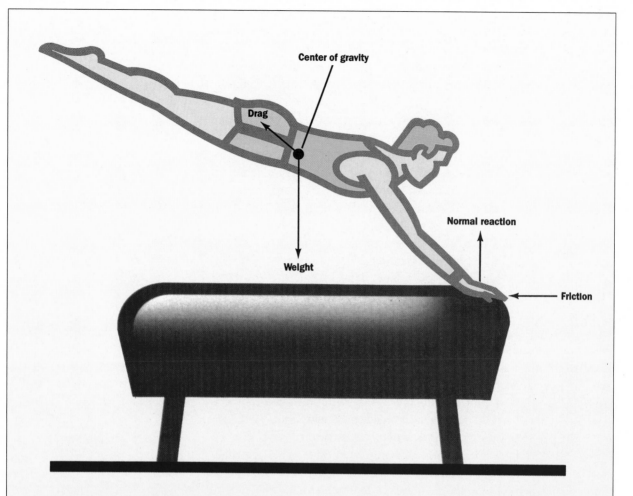

Center of gravity

Drag

Weight

Normal reaction

Friction

Forces That Affect Motion

Your body is always subject to forces that can
cause it to shift position or remain stable, to
accelerate or decelerate. In everyday life, you
are usually unaware of the forces acting upon
you, but as soon as you begin practicing
unfamiliar movements, such as gymnastic
routines, these forces become noticeable.

The most constant force is gravity, which
exerts a pull that keeps you rooted to the planet.
At the point where your body is in contact with
the ground or with some other object, like the
vaulting horse in the illustration, two other
forces come into play: friction and normal
reaction. Friction is the resistance that a moving
object encounters when it comes into contact
with the surface of another object. Normal

reaction is the term for Newton's law that for
every action, there is an equal and opposite
reaction. This means that the vaulting horse is
pushing upward on the gymnast to the same
degree that he is pushing downward on it.
Finally, motion is slowed by drag, a function of
acceleration through the flow of air, which
opposes your forward momentum.

The relative strength of these forces varies,
depending on the activity and the speed of your
movement. In the illustration, this relative
strength can be gauged by the length of the
arrows. By analyzing forces systematically,
trainers and coaches can help gymnasts and
other athletes refine their techniques to improve
performance.

activity are too closely related to separate them into elements that can be practiced on their own.

On the other hand, studies show that the best way to learn a gymnastic or dance movement involving steps that are relatively independent of each other is to break the exercise down into simpler fundamentals and practice these elements until you can perform them correctly. Research demonstrates that the more meaningful the practice movements are, the easier they are to learn.

In other words, as you practice individual dance or gymnastic programs, you should separate them into segments that are easy to practice, but not into such small and insignificant parts that it becomes difficult to relate them to the exercise as a whole. You must be able to keep in mind just how the movement you are practicing fits into the larger organization of the routine.

In what ways do gymnastics and dance movement improve your physical fitness?
Both gymnastics and dance promote strength and flexibility, and, when performed intensively for a prolonged period of time, they also build up your aerobic endurance. A typical gymnastic routine almost always involves supporting your body weight with your hands and arms in a way that builds muscle power. In fact, most gymnastic coaches believe that all strength-building calisthenics, such as push-ups and sit-ups, are actually gymnastic movements.

Gymnastic activities develop flexibility because they involve moving and holding your body in positions that encourage your muscles to stretch farther than they do during everyday movements or other kinds of exercises. Many people who exercise frequently avoid doing a regular program of stretching because they consider it to be a boring activity. However, a simple gymnastic routine incorporates stretching in a variety of ways that are more interesting and enjoyable than many other exercise programs.

How to Design Your Own Program

If you have never practiced graceful movements, you should first determine what level of gymnastic activity you can perform safely. The questions and self-assessment tests here and on the following pages are designed to help you measure your strength and flexibility. After answering the questions and taking the tests, turn to the Guide to the Exercises on pages 20-21, and find the exercises for which you are qualified. Do not attempt movements that are too advanced for you. For exercisers at all levels, gymnastics can be dangerous if you do movements that are too difficult or if you try complicated ones without the aid of an experienced spotter or assistant.

How agile are you?

1 Are you naturally graceful?

Everyone has at least some natural agility that can be developed, and there is no one who is so hopelessly uncoordinated that an exercise program cannot help. Of course, it is true that some people have superior potential for agility, just as others are born with the potential to be artists. The fact remains that people with the innate talent to paint must learn painting techniques, and those with inborn potential for agility must practice whatever movements they need for their sport or exercise. Gymnasts must practice their routines over and over to get them right, just as professional athletes must hone their skills continually.

2 Have you reached a plateau in your fitness program?

Whether you lift weights or do an aerobic activity such as running to stay in shape, you may sometimes find that you reach a plateau that prevents your fitness from progressing. At some point in your training, it may seem impossible to improve your race times or increase the amount of weight you are able to lift, no matter how hard you push yourself. When this happens, switching to a new type of exercise program may help. By building upper-body strength, increasing your flexibility and enhancing your body awareness, gymnastic exercises like the activities shown in this book can provide you with a fresh perspective for your workouts. Performing these exercises can help you enter a new phase of training in your regular sport, and make it possible for you to progress beyond a plateau as a result.

3 Do you get bored with stretching?

Stretching to stay flexible can be a dull activity. For this reason, many people neglect stretching even though flexibility is vital for fitness and necessary for maintaining the range of motion of your joints. Performing slow, steady gymnastic moves, such as the exercises in the beginning of Chapter Two, offers a way of stretching that is fun and beneficial. If you do them while listening to music, these rhythmic exercises can not only help you develop flexibility, they also promote strength and body awareness. The partner exercises in Chapter Four will extend your range of motion by allowing you to stretch farther and in ways you would not be able to stretch by yourself.

4 Can tumbling ability improve your performance and agility in other sports?

Yes. Tumbling not only improves your sense of balance and body awareness generally, it also helps you develop the ability to fall safely. When you know how to fall correctly, your performance in sports in which falling is nearly inevitable, like ice hockey, skating and football, will improve. Since agility is usually increased when you are appropriately relaxed, not being afraid to fall will make you more agile. Furthermore, if you know how to fall safely, you are much less likely to be injured when you do fall.

5 Are these exercises safe?

While many of the exercises in this book are meant for you to perform on your own — for example, the balances in Chapter Two — it is wise to have a spotter nearby when you perform the tumbling exercises shown in Chapter Three. Gymnastic movements can be difficult, even dangerous, if you do them incorrectly and without the proper preparation. (For tips on spotting, see page 95.) You should also protect yourself by determining your readiness to try a particular movement by taking the self-assessment tests on pages 18-19, and by making certain that you have mastered the elementary exercises before trying the more difficult routines in Chapters Three and Four.

6 Should you work with a partner?

Yes, for some exercises. Interacting with a partner adds another dimension to your development of agility, making you aware of how your body moves in relation to an another person's. You can also work with a partner to increase your upper- and lower-body strength, using each other's body weight for resistance, and to enhance your ability to balance, creating graceful movements together, as shown in Chapter Four.

NEGATIVE SIT-UP: From a seated position, with your knees raised and feet flat on the floor, slowly lower yourself halfway to the floor *(right).* Hold this position for as long as possible. Scoring: Excellent: 25 seconds. Good: 15. Fair: 5. Poor: less than 5. **PUSH-UPS:** Do as many push-ups as you can — either the classic extended-leg version or this easier variation, with your knees on the floor *(below right).* Scoring: Excellent: 25. Good: 15. Fair: 5. Poor: fewer than 5.

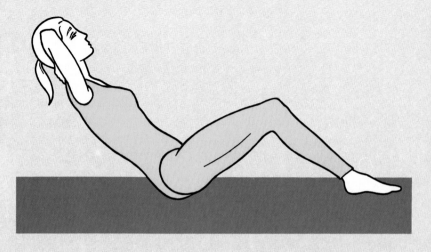

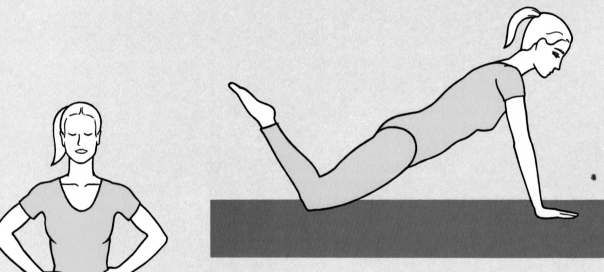

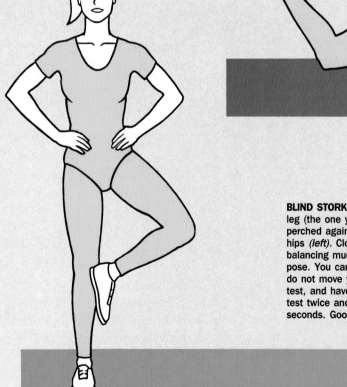

BLIND STORK: Stand on a hard surface on your dominant leg (the one you would kick a ball with), with your other foot perched against the opposite knee and your hands on your hips *(left).* Close your eyes (keeping them open makes balancing much easier) and time how long you can hold the pose. You can sway and shift your position so long as you do not move your supporting foot. Wear sneakers for this test, and have a friend time you with a stopwatch. Take the test twice and record your best time. Scoring: Excellent: 50 seconds. Good: 30. Fair: 10. Poor: less than 5.

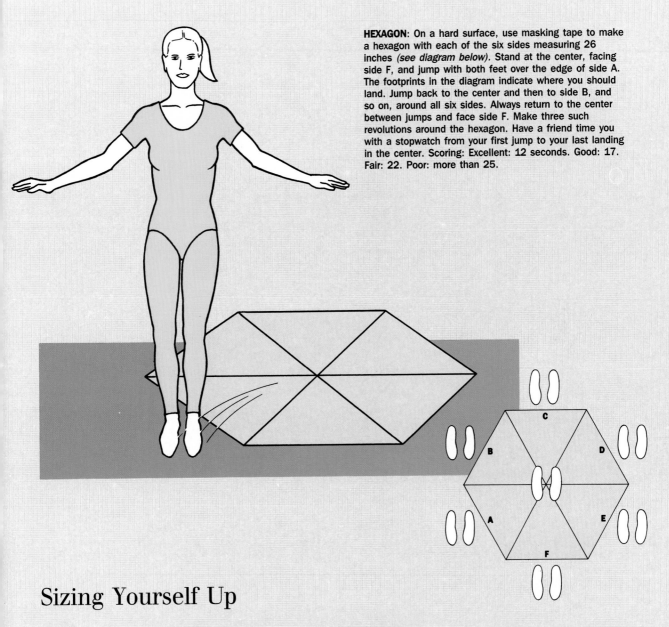

HEXAGON: On a hard surface, use masking tape to make a hexagon with each of the six sides measuring 26 inches (see diagram below). Stand at the center, facing side F, and jump with both feet over the edge of side A. The footprints in the diagram indicate where you should land. Jump back to the center and then to side B, and so on, around all six sides. Always return to the center between jumps and face side F. Make three such revolutions around the hexagon. Have a friend time you with a stopwatch from your first jump to your last landing in the center. Scoring: Excellent: 12 seconds. Good: 17. Fair: 22. Poor: more than 25.

Sizing Yourself Up

The routines in this book require balance, strength and agility. Before you begin, take the following four self-assessment tests to find out your present skill level. If your skill level is poor or fair, begin with the introductory exercises indicated on pages 20-21. If your level is good or excellent, start with the movements in the beginner category; you will probably progress quickly to the intermediate level if you have some gymnastic or dance experience.

The push-up and negative sit-up tests (opposite) measure the strength of your upper body and abdomen. When performing the push-ups, be sure to keep your back straight and do them smoothly and at a moderate pace until you cannot complete another repetition.

The Blind Stork test (opposite, bottom) assesses your ability to balance. When you take the test, keep your center of gravity positioned over your supporting foot.

The Hexagon test (above) tests your coordination and your agility. Make sure you take this test on a level floor. Do the test several times and figure your score from your best performance. However, do each test trial immediately after the previous one. Taking a break will allow you to become too familiar with it.

Getting Started

When choosing your exercises from this guide, you should always use caution and stay well within your capabilities. After taking the self-assessment tests on pages 18-19, if you are still unsure of where to begin, perform the introductory exercises. Then you can use your experience with those exercises to determine your ability to progress to the more advanced movements.

There are several reasons for being conservative in your choice of tumbling routines: Attempting to do gymnastic exercises for which you are unprepared can be dangerous as well as being of limited benefit to your physical fitness. You must first master the fundamental skills that are needed for an exercise, since you may not be able to perform a more advanced movement without risk of an injury.

It is also necessary to have an experienced spotter on hand when you do the more advanced exercises. These more difficult movements should be approached the same way you would take a swim in the ocean — never do them alone. For a quick review of basic spotting techniques, refer to the box on page 95.

Do not rush your way through these exercises. For best results, limit your program to learning one or two basic skills at a time. If you try to learn too much at once, it will slow your mastery of necessary individual skills, and it may cause excess fatigue, which could also hamper your progress.

A Guide to the Exercises

INTRODUCTORY

These exercises require little training and preparation and can be performed by virtually anyone who does not have a limiting physical condition, such as a bad back. The movements are designed to develop strength and flexibility. If you need to improve both capacities, begin with these exercises. Master them before progressing to any other section of exercises.

pages 26-29, 36-45, 61, 96-97, 99, 106

INTERMEDIATE

The intermediate movements require some tumbling skill. They range in difficulty from a basic backbend to a cartwheel. While the safety of these exercises increases when you have someone to assist or spot you, it is still possible to suffer an injury if you perform them incorrectly or if you lack the necessary strength and flexibility.

pages 50-51, 54-55, 62-65, 72-79, 82-83, 88-89, 107-109, 116-121

DIFFICULT

These exercises should only be attempted after you have become proficient in tumbling technique. Performed properly, the positions will challenge the novice gymnast who wishes to enhance his or her acrobatic skill. After you have developed a high degree of strength and flexibility, try the movements with a partner who knows how to spot.

pages 70-71, 84-85, 90-91, 111, 122-123

BEGINNER

The exercises in this category are slightly more challenging than the introductory ones. These movements demand a certain amount of strength and flexibility, and they improve these attributes and enhance your ability to balance in various poses. Being proficient at these exercises is a prerequisite to performing the intermediate and difficult gymnastics exercises in this book.

pages 30-35, 46-49, 52-53, 60, 66-69, 80-81, 86-87, 98, 100-105, 112, 115

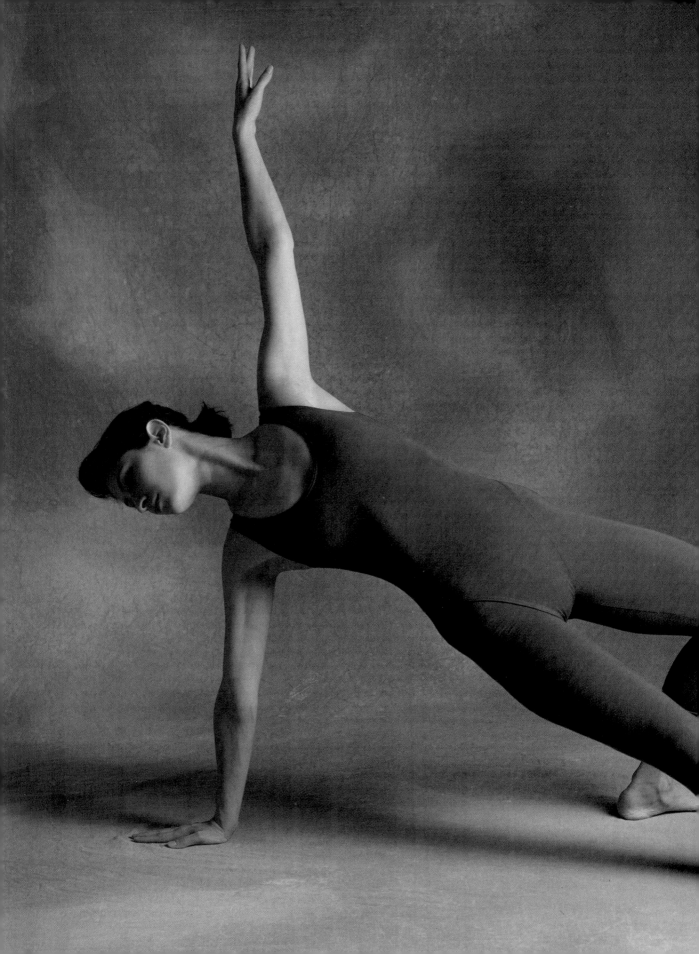

CHAPTER TWO

Finding Your Center

Routines that build form

Gymnastics and dance are meant to be performed for an audience; they are designed to demonstrate the graceful body in motion. Consequently, all serious gymnasts and dancers make form their primary consideration (many practice their routines in front of large mirrors). In contrast, people who engage in most other sports and aerobic activities often focus almost exclusively on endurance or strength; graceful movement and body awareness are of secondary importance. For example, many runners and bicyclists are more concerned with how far and fast they can travel rather than how they look as they exercise.

The fact is, even if you ignore your form when you exercise or compete, you will inevitably develop a style of movement. A haphazardly developed style may well be awkward and inefficient, since it is dictated by unconscious habits. Runners, for instance, often tense their backs and shoulders, wasting energy that could be used for speed or endurance. Many bicyclists favor one side or lean forward

23

excessively as they pedal, making them use extra force to compensate for being off balance. Their unconscious movement habits impede their effectiveness as athletes.

Developing grace and precision in your movement can give you increased control and make better use of your energy. This efficiency ensures that you minimize wasted effort — that your muscles do not work against one another. And it also helps prevent injury: You are less likely to pull muscles or overload tendons if your form is correct. Properly performed movements result in the safest and most even distribution of the bodily stress involved in any activity.

The exercises in this chapter are designed to increase your body awareness while they develop your flexibility and strength. Derived from basic dance and gymnastic movements, the unusual motions involved in these exercises force you to control and monitor your body position carefully as you proceed step by step. When you begin, it is important to focus on maintaining proper form and using the appropriate muscles for the sequence of movements. As you practice for a period of weeks, you will find that the motions become easier and feel more comfortable to perform.

Your gradually increasing familiarity with the exercises will be the result of your body's ability to incorporate learned movements into your system of unconscious muscular control. Just as you learned to balance on a bicycle, you will learn to perform these exercises by directly experiencing the motions they require. As you practice, you will learn what is necessary to complete the proper motions and recognize how your body should feel as you do them.

Be sure to warm up sufficiently before beginning these exercises. The movements may seem more strenuous than they appear at first glance. Any time you twist your torso and extremities or move any part of your body through a range of motion that you are unaccustomed to, you may subject your muscles and connective tissues to a substantial amount of stress. That can be harmful if you have not warmed up beforehand. In fact, some of the most common injuries gymnasts suffer are strained or pulled muscles as a result of performing without adequate preparation.

Warming up means just that — raising your internal body temperature as well as increasing your heart rate. Ideally your exercise session should start with at least five minutes of an activity such as jogging or pedaling a stationary bicycle. However, you can warm up by performing the exercises on pages 26-35 very slowly and gently. Do each one two times, and do not expect yourself to stretch to your maximum capacity right away. The warm-up activity can raise your internal body temperature to more than 100 degrees F. Warm muscles stretch more easily than cold ones do, and increased circulation will provide them with the energy they need to do the exercises. A sufficiently warmed-up nervous system can transmit impulses faster from brain and reflex centers in the spine to the muscles throughout the body.

Movement Terms

Gymnasts and dancers use a number of terms to describe the movements and positions they perform. The following terms apply to routines shown in this book:

◆ BATTEMENT A movement of the foot in any direction done from a standing position, with the toes pointed.

◆ DEMI-PLIÉ A knee bend done with the back straight and the feet flat on the floor, used for taking off and landing in jumps.

◆ LUNGE A standing position with one leg to the front, knee bent, and the other leg stretched out backward. The weight is on the front leg, the body inclined forward.

◆ PLIÉ A knee bend with the knees bent over the toes, deep enough so that the thighs are parallel to the floor.

◆ RELEVÉ A rise onto the balls of the feet from a standing position, done with the back straight.

◆ ROLL A complete revolution of the body on the floor from a stance on the feet. Rolls are done in a tucked position over a curved spine, forward, backward or sideways. They are sometimes confused with somersaults.

◆ SCALE A standing balance performed on one leg. A scale can be done on the floor, on another gymnast or on a piece of apparatus, with the raised leg and upper body parallel to the floor.

◆ SOMERSAULT A complete revolution of the body, forward or backward, in the air.

◆ SPOTTING Help from an onlooker when doing a gymnastic exercise to prevent the gymnast from injury, either by means of the spotter's hands guiding the gymnast through a movement, or by the spotter's readiness to intervene at any point, if necessary.

◆ TURNOUT The capacity to rotate the legs outward in the hip sockets while maintaining proper body alignment, so that the toes point out to the sides, and the knees are positioned directly over the toes.

When you first perform the exercises in this chapter, you should pay special attention to keeping your body straight and relaxed. Avoid hunching your shoulders or otherwise straining. Except where otherwise directed, keep your buttocks tucked in and avoid an arched back. Work slowly and thoughtfully, focusing on the muscles that are stretched or contracted for each motion. Stretch only as far as it is comfortable for you. Do not push yourself to the point of feeling pain in your muscles, tendons or joints. With practice, you should become stronger and more flexible.

To make your exercise session more enjoyable, and to help yourself remain relaxed, consider doing it as you listen to music. You should also breathe comfortably at all times. Be careful not to hold your breath, since it can prevent blood from returning to the heart, and also cause abdominal cramps. Do the exercises at moderate speed and relax in between each set of movements until you are accustomed to performing them easily. If you cannot do a sequence completely, do as much of it as you can, or break it down into component parts.

On the Floor/1

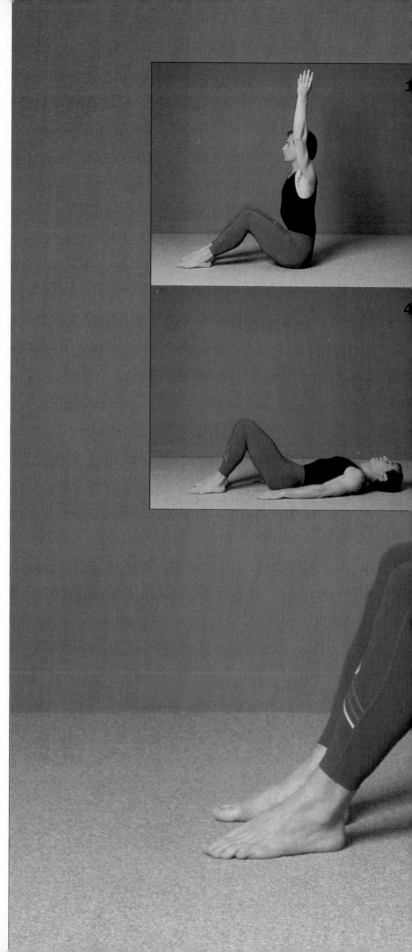

After you warm up with a brief aerobic routine, perform the following exercises in the order shown to develop your abdominal and arm strength, and extend the flexibility of your back and legs. It is especially important to perform the floor exercises on these two pages and on pages 28-35 slowly and smoothly, without bouncing movements. If you rush, you may do them too quickly and easily. Some of these poses are difficult to achieve and hold when performed slowly — but the slower you proceed, the more strength you will develop.

A mat is not required to do the floor exercises that follow, but you will be more comfortable performing them on a rug or other padded surface. You can do the exercises barefoot since you will not be jumping or bouncing. If you are barefoot, your feet can grip the floor without slipping.

All these floor exercises will develop strength in your abdomen. The exercise shown on these first two pages also provides a good stretch for your back. The exercise on pages 28-29 involves stretching the lower back and the back of the leg, which may be difficult to do if you are not very flexible. The last stage of the exercise on pages 32-33 and the exercise on pages 34-35 require a great deal of arm strength. If you cannot complete the exercise, do as much of it as possible.

Sit with your knees bent, feet flat on the floor and arms straight over your head (1). With palms up, reach your hands forward as you slowly roll downward from your spine, vertebra by vertebra (2,3), until your back, head and hands are on the floor (4). Raise your buttocks slowly, tail bone first (5), keeping your shoulders and feet on the floor (6) until you form a bridge and your thighs are almost parallel to the ground (bottom right). Return to the starting position slowly by reversing the steps.

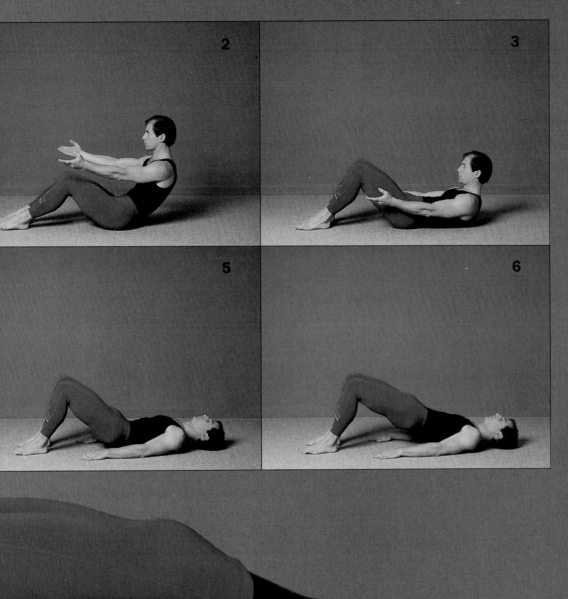

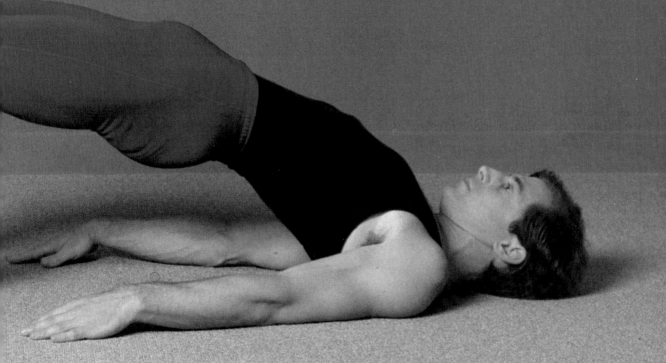

On the Floor/2

Lie on your back and use your hands to bring your right knee to your chest (1). Hold for 15 seconds, then let go of your leg. Place your hands on the floor with your arms straight out to the sides, your right thigh perpendicular and your lower right leg parallel to the floor (2). Keeping your upper body as straight as possible, bring your right knee down to the floor on the left side of your body (3). Hold for 15 seconds. Bring your right leg back to the central position and grip the back of your leg just above the ankle (4). Straightening your leg as much as possible, gently pull the ankle close to your face without straining (5). Hold for 15 seconds. Slowly lower your right leg and hands to the floor (6). Repeat with your other leg.

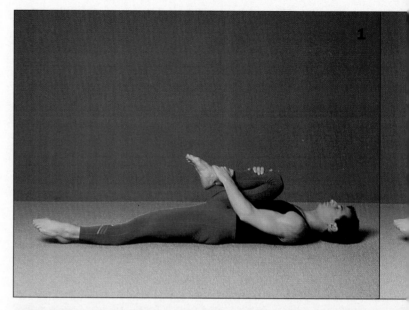

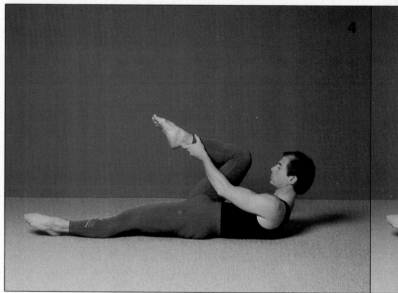

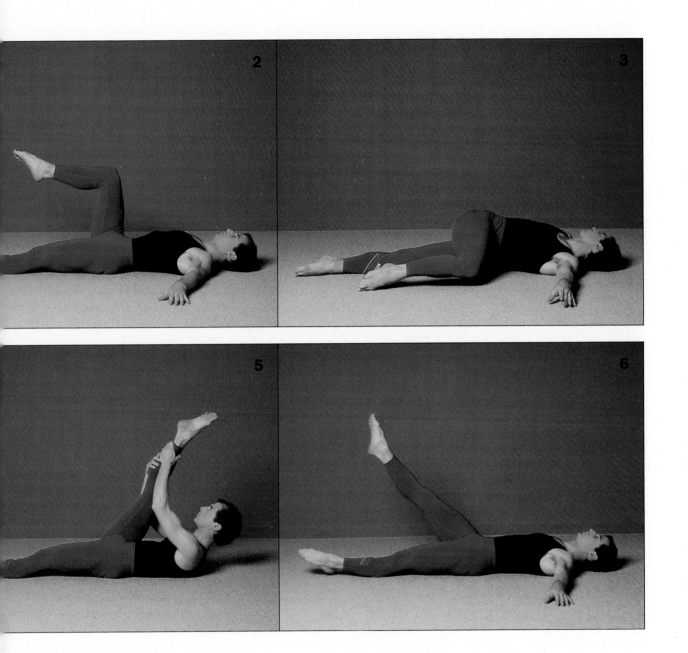

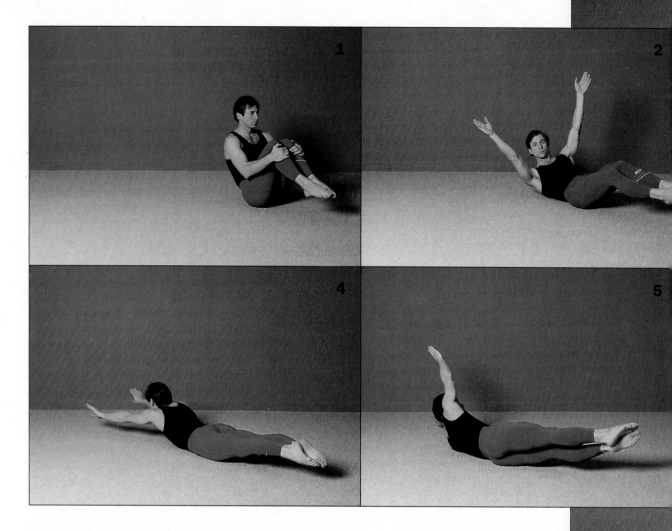

On the Floor/3

Sit on the floor, balanced on your buttocks, with your knees bent, feet off the floor and your hands gripping your knees (1). Let go of your knees, slowly straighten your legs and lift your hands over your head as you roll to the right (2). With a straight body, hands over your head, continue rolling to your right (3). Keeping your body straight, roll over onto your stomach, with your knees, lower legs, chest and arms off the floor, if possible (4). Continue to roll on to your left hip (5) and then onto your back, lifting your legs only as necessary to keep the lower back flat on the floor (6). Sit up, bringing your knees to your chest (7), and continue until you are in the starting position.

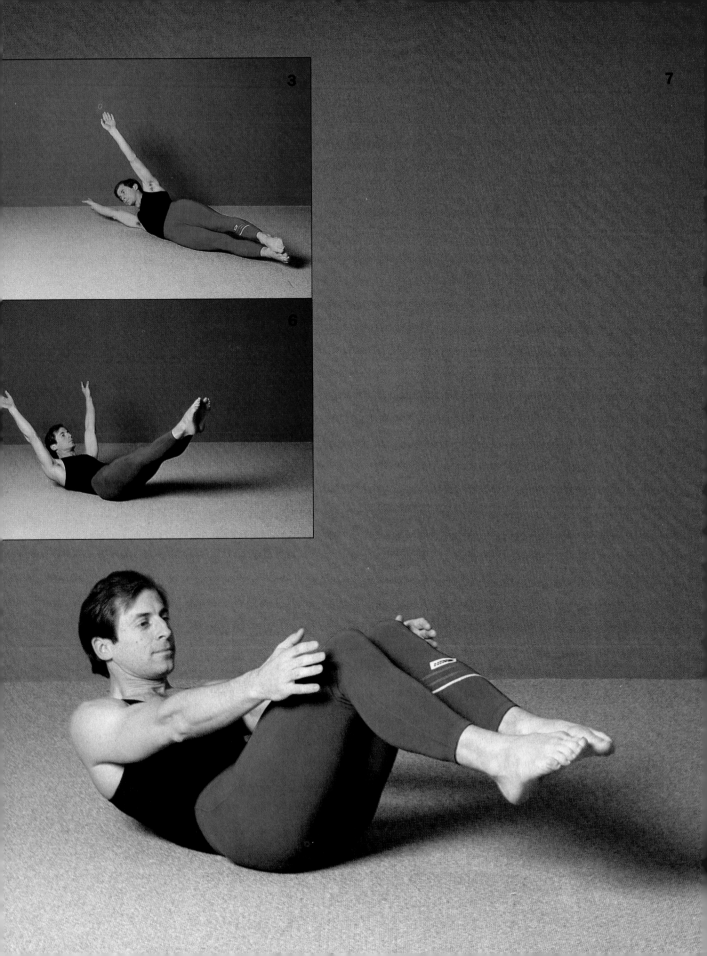

On the Floor/4

Lie on your stomach with arms bent in the push-up position. Raise your head and bring your chest up, supporting your upper body with your hands on the floor (1). Lift your stomach off the floor and round your spine while tucking your buttocks until you are on all fours (2). Straighten your legs, put your feet flat on the floor, keep your arms straight and form a triangle with your buttocks as the highest point (3). Keeping your neck stretched toward the floor, roll forward through the spine in a wavelike motion that brings your head through your arms (4). Slowly bring your lower body to the floor, keeping your arms straight and your chest up (5). Bend your arms, roll downward through your stomach and chest to the push-up position. Then lie on your stomach with arms straight in front of you and lower legs off the floor (6). Lower your chin to the floor, bend your knees and reach back and grasp your feet (7). Lift your head as far as possible (8). Release your feet carefully, lower your head, straighten your legs, put your hands on the floor and assume the push-up position (9). Perform five to 10 push-ups (10).

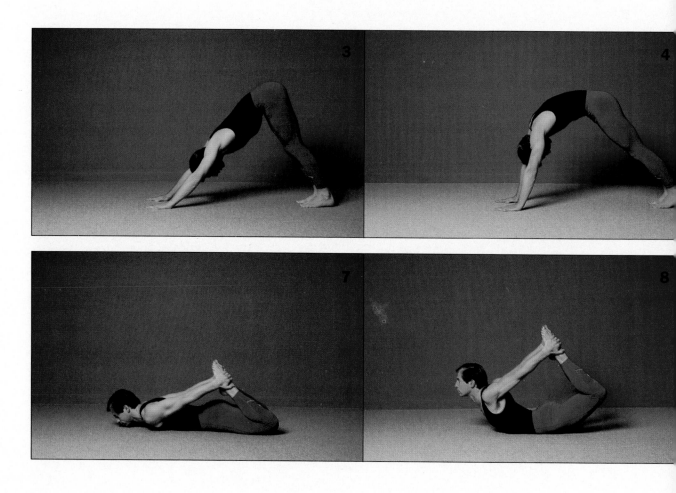

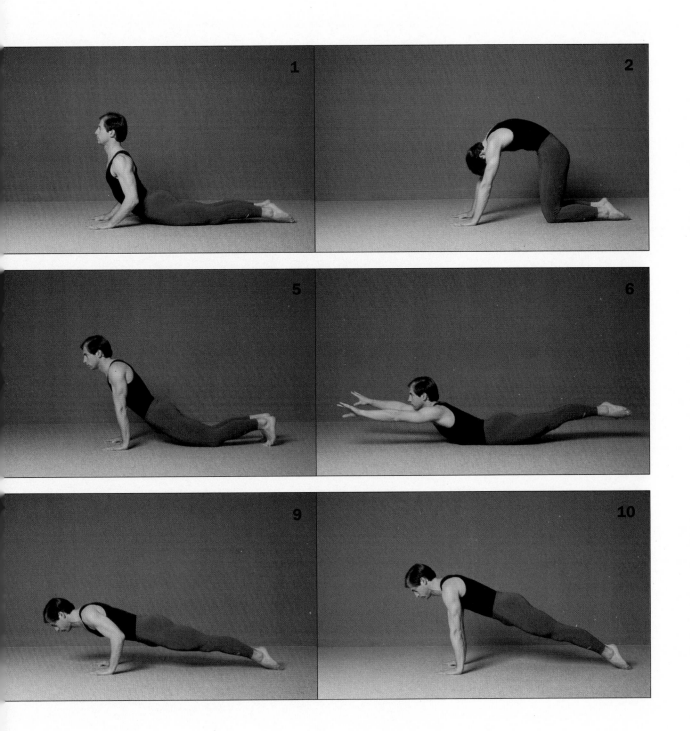

On the Floor/5

Sit on the floor with your right leg extended and your left leg bent with your left foot flat on the floor. Put your right hand on the floor slightly behind you and your left arm straight in front of you, palm up (1). Shift your weight to the right, raising your left hand above and your buttocks off the floor as you turn your body (2). Continue turning to your right as you bring your left hand upward (3). Finish with your upper body sideways and parallel to the floor, your left hand straight up (4). Reverse the exercise steps and return to starting position. Repeat to the other side.

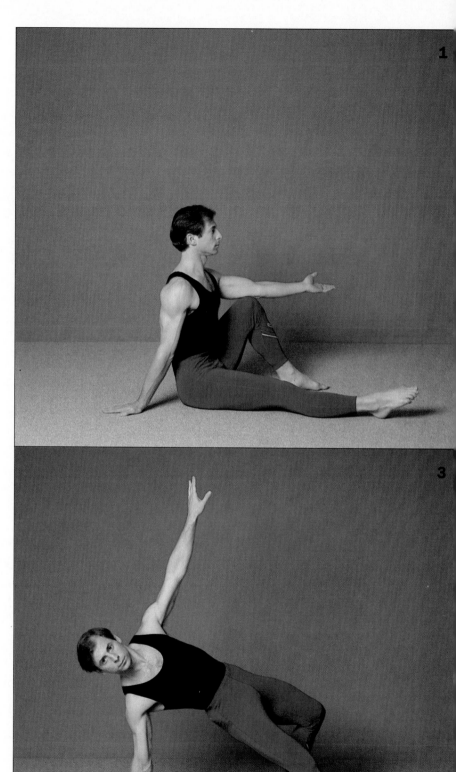

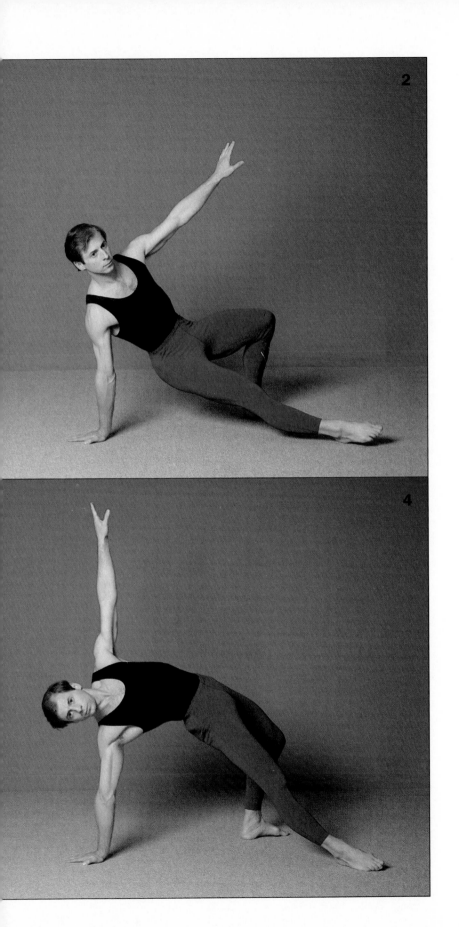

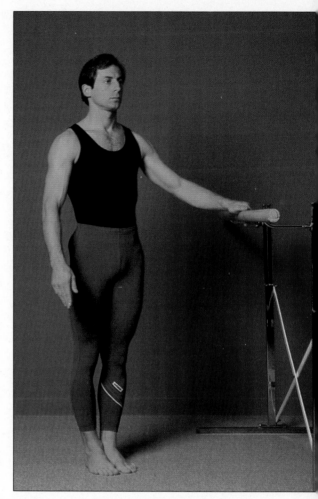

With your right hand at your side, hold the barre with your left hand. Place your feet together pointing straight ahead *(near right).* Bending your knees, slowly lower your body, keeping your back perpendicular to the floor *(center).* Return to the starting position and press upward on the balls of your feet *(far right);* then return again. Repeat five times.

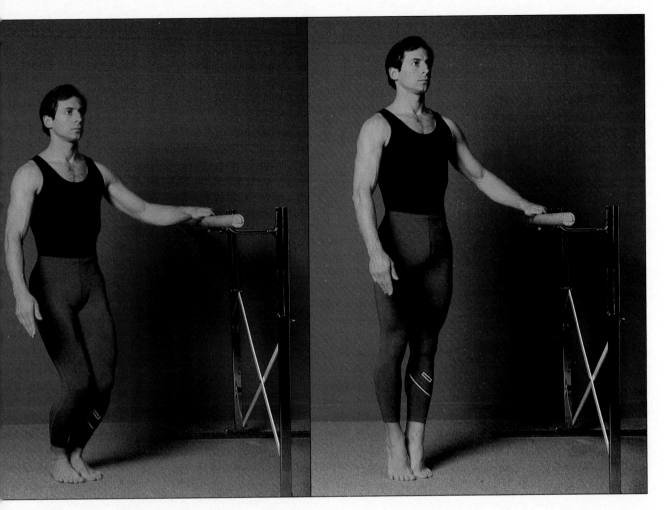

At the Barre/1

Perform the following exercises to develop your sense of body alignment. You must watch yourself closely to maintain the positions shown precisely. As you become familiar with the movements, you will find your body beginning to move into the correct positions with ease.

A barre is simply a support rod used by dancers to balance themselves while they practice dance poses and movements. When you practice movements at home, you do not need a specially made barre. You can use any stable piece of furniture, railing or steady shelf at the appropriate height for your body as long as it is secured firmly.

The barre exercises on pages 38-39 are done from basic ballet foot positions, which are called first (heels together and feet turned outward as pictured at the top of pages 38-39), and second (feet apart and turned outward as shown on the bottom of pages 38-39).

When assuming these positions, proper posture and body stance are the most important considerations and the most common source of mistakes. Be sure to keep your knees over your feet. Try not to let your buttocks protrude, but resist the urge to tuck them in excessively. Either position will look unnatural and forced, and will make the exercises harder to do.

Demi-plié, the ballet posture that presents the most problems for beginners, is shown in the center of the bottom sequence on pages 38-39. When you are in this posture, your back should remain perpendicular to the floor at all times; resist the impulse to lean forward, a common error.

After performing these ballet positions, you should hold the shoulder and rear leg stretches shown on pages 40-41 for 30 seconds to a minute before doing the simple ballet leg movements shown on pages 42-43. These stretches will loosen any tightness in your legs and shoulders and make it easier for you to extend your legs.

At the Barre/2

With your right hand at your side, hold the barre with your left hand. Keep your heels together and point your toes to the sides so that your feet form an angle of approximately 120 degrees (1). Keeping your back straight, bend your knees and lower yourself without lifting your heels off the floor (2). Straighten your knees and move upward on your toes as high as possible (3); then come down. Move your feet apart about one or two feet and point your toes to the sides at a 120-degree angle (4). Bend your knees and lower your body while keeping your back straight (5). Return to the starting position but with your feet still apart and raise yourself on your toes as high as possible; then come down.

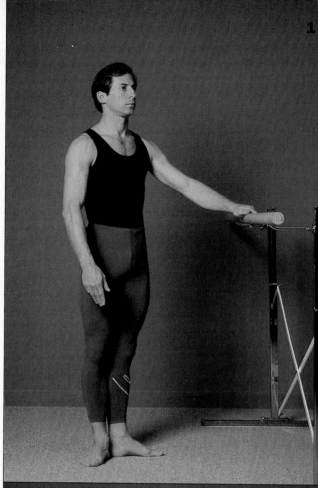

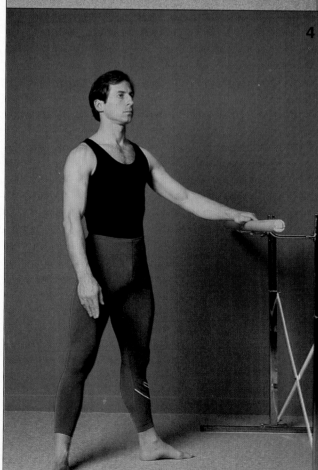

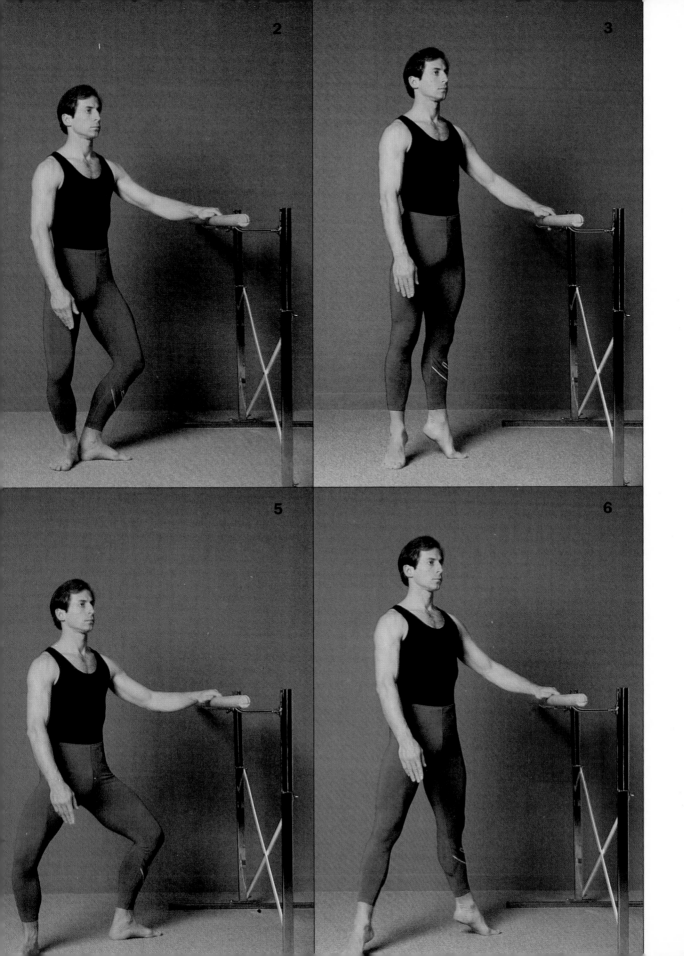

At the Barre/3

Stand about four feet from the barre.
Keeping your arms and legs straight,
grasp the barre with both hands and drop
your head as far as possible. Relax and
feel the stretch in your shoulders *(right)*.
Hold this position for 30-60 seconds.
Keeping your head between your arms,
lift your head and shoulders until you feel
a stretch in your upper back and chest
(bottom right). Hold for 30-60 seconds.

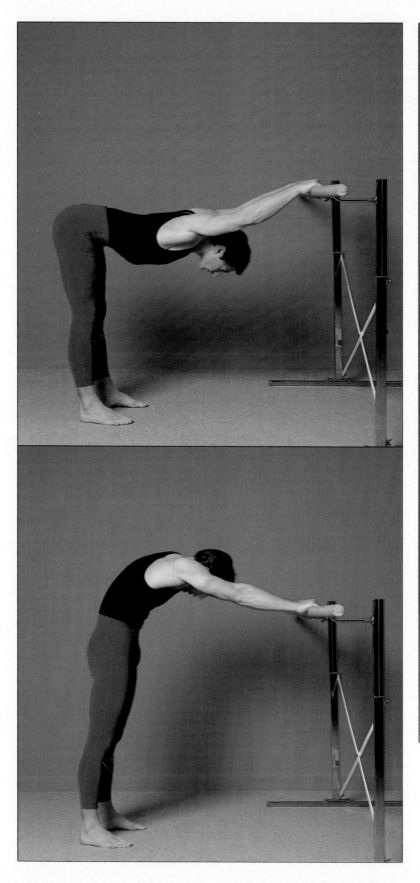

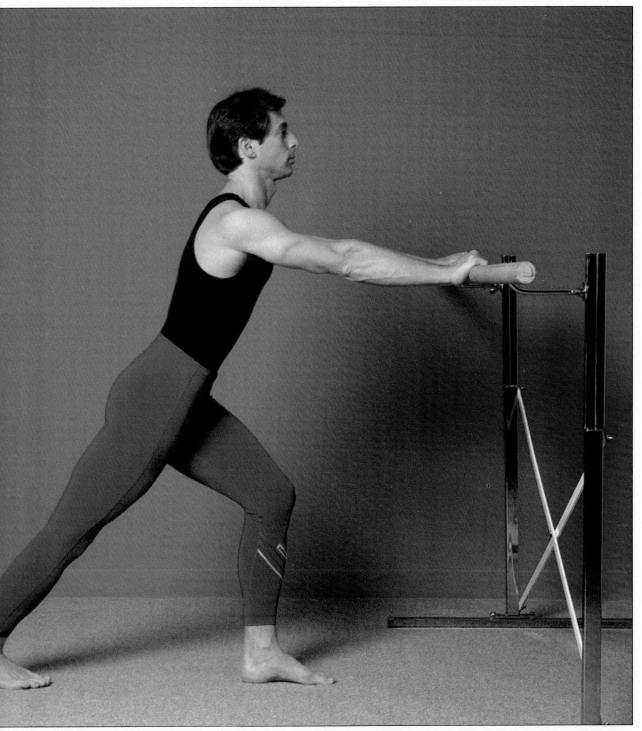

Hold the barre with both hands, draw your left knee forward and extend your right leg backward in a parallel position. Keep your right knee straight *(above)*. Hold for 30-60 seconds. Repeat with your other leg.

At the Barre/4

Hold the barre with your left hand. Extend your right arm out to the side for balance while you stand with your heels together and feet pointed out at a 120-degree angle (1). Keeping your right leg as straight as possible, lift your right foot off the floor and bring it up as high as you can as you point your toes forward (2). Hold for a moment, then return it to the floor. Raise your right leg out to the side (3) and hold for a moment. Return it to the floor. Raise your right foot backward (4) and hold for a moment. Return it to the floor. Repeat with your left foot.

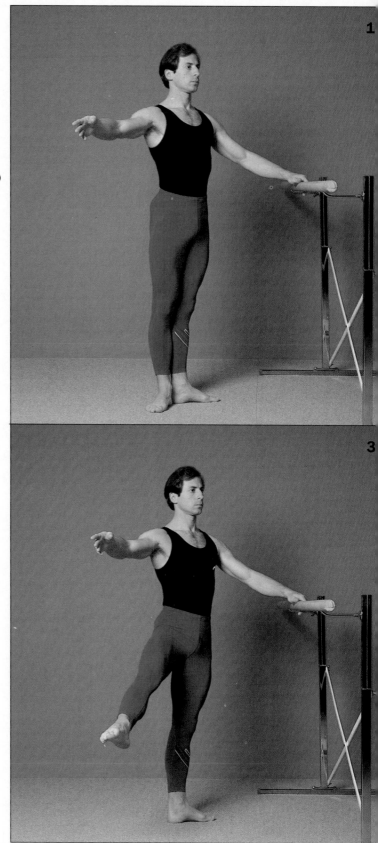

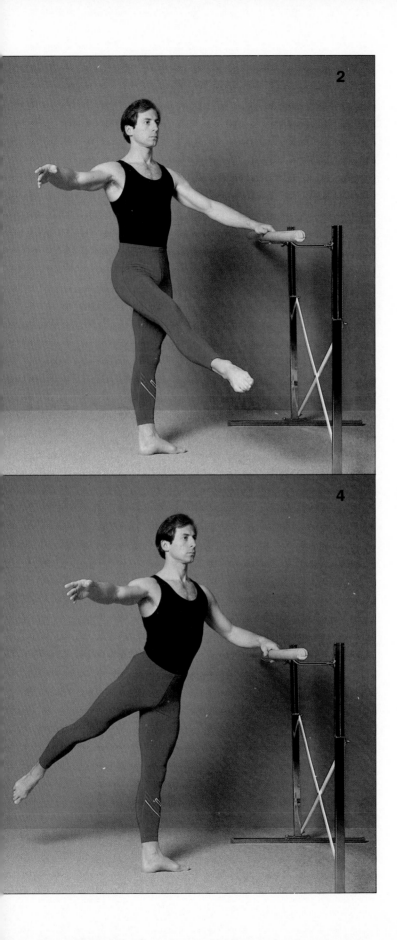

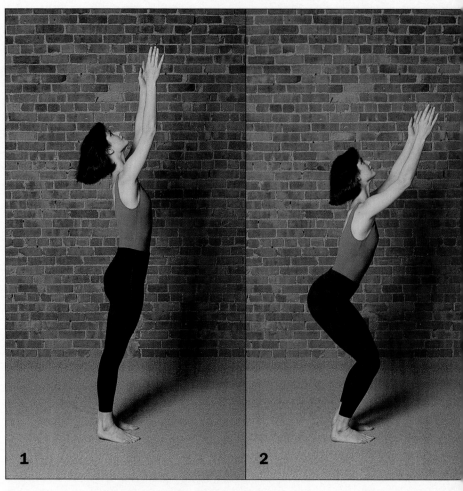

Balance and Coordination/1

The coordination and balance exercises on these two pages and on pages 46-55 will add another dimension to the skills you have developed in the preceding exercises. While the earlier routines develop strength, precision of body placement and flexibility, the following exercises will help you combine these with an increased ability to balance in unusual positions and maneuver your body.

Strive for fluidity of motion that is smooth rather than jerky and abrupt. For instance, when you do the arm swings on these two pages, or the foot-to-hand movement on pages 46-47, you may be tempted to over-reach the illustrated positions ballistically, using a sudden reach or kick. While it is true that such ballistic movements will help you reach further, they will also increase your chance of injury.

The exercises on pages 48-55 require you to balance on one foot. Before performing them, be sure you can stand on one foot unaided for at least 30 seconds. You may find this easier if you focus your gaze on a point at eye level about 10 feet in front of you. If you have trouble performing them, use a barre or a balancing aid.

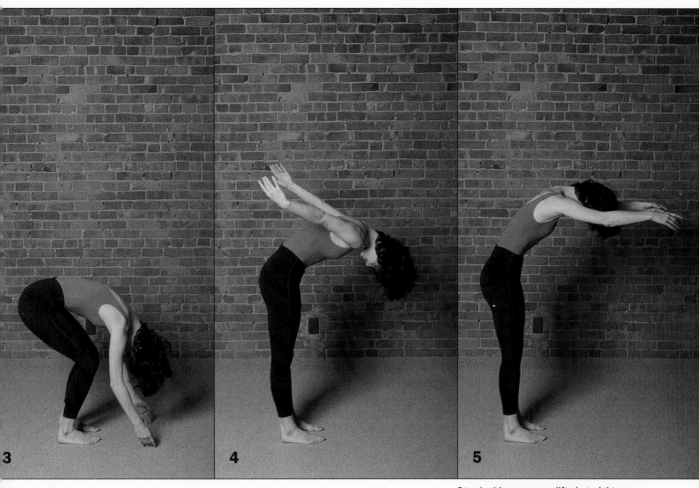

3 **4** **5**

Stand with your arms lifted straight up
(1). While bending your knees, arch your
back slightly, lean forward and start to
swing your hands to the floor (2). Reach
downward to brush your hands along the
floor (3). Continue swinging your hands
behind you as you raise upward. Contract
your stomach and straighten your knees
(4). As you start to reverse the movement, swing your arms forward (5) and
return to the starting position as you
straighten your back.

Balance and Coordination/2

Stand with your left arm extended in front of you and your right arm relaxed at your side *(right)*. Bring your left leg backward while balancing on your right foot *(center)*. Swing your left leg forward, trying to bring it as close as possible to your hand, while keeping your foot flexed *(far right)*. Repeat five times and then switch legs.

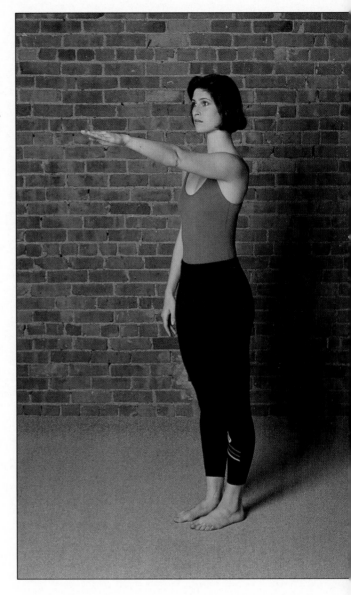

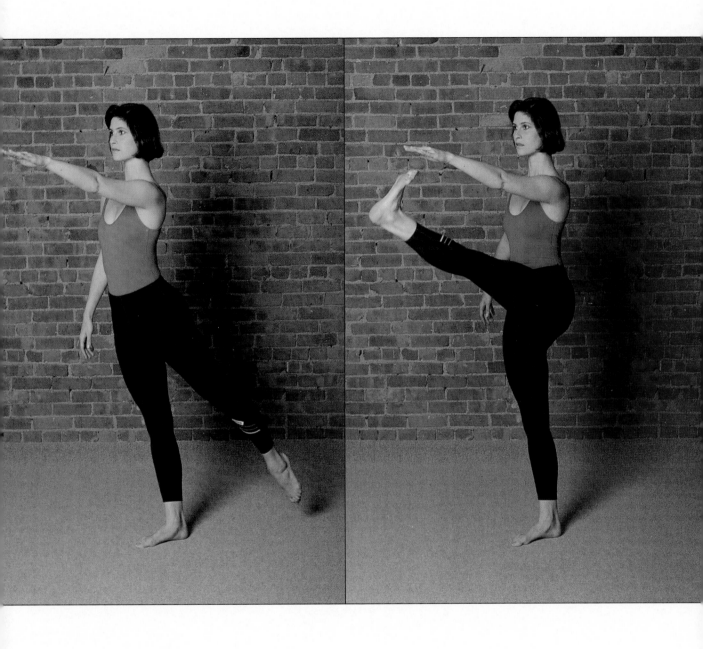

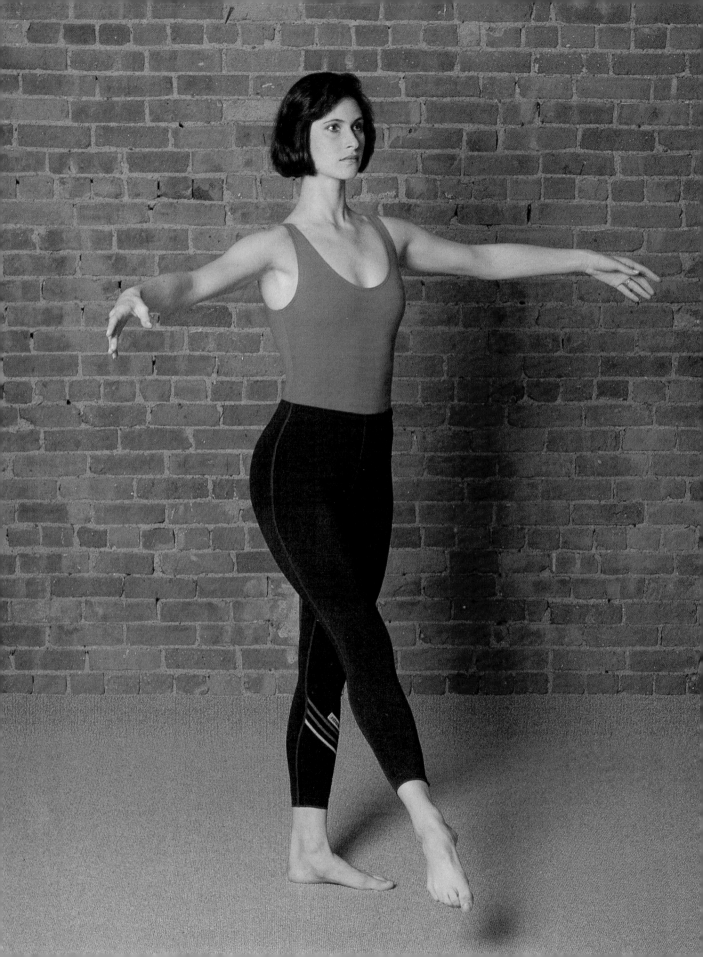

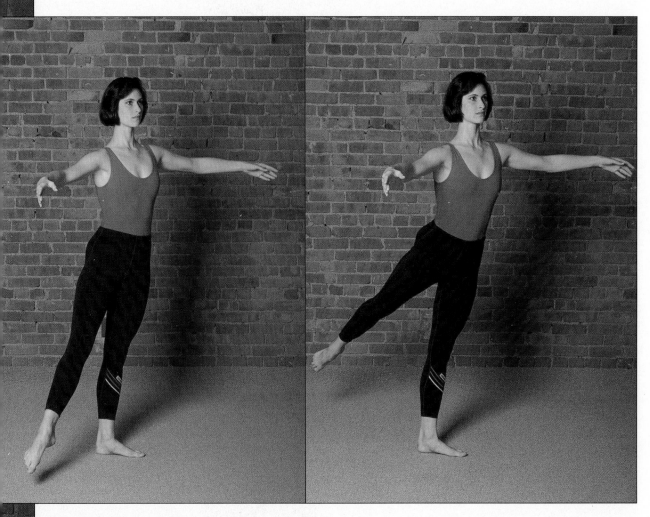

Balance and Coordination/3

Stand with your arms out to the sides for balance. Bring your right leg forward as far as possible with your knee straight *(left)*. Hold this position for a moment, then return it to the floor. Raise your right leg to the right and hold for a moment *(above)*. Raise your right foot backward as far as possible and hold for a moment *(above right)*, then return it to the floor. Repeat with your other leg.

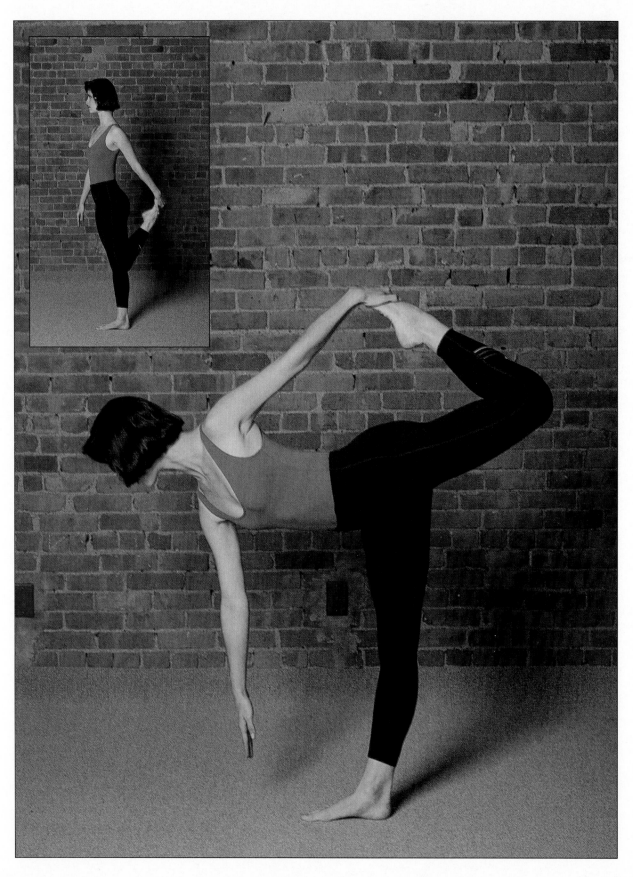

Balance and Coordination/4

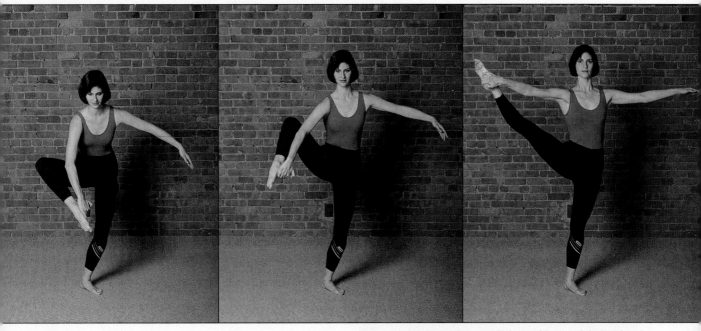

From a standing position, reach down with your right hand and hold the inside of your right heel *(above left)*. Straighten up as you bring your leg to the side and extend your left arm for balance *(center)*. Stand erect with your right leg raised to the side as high as possible, your left arm parallel to the floor *(right)*. Hold this position for as long as possible. Repeat with your other leg.

While standing, reach backward and grasp your left foot with your left hand, lifting it so that your knee forms about a 45-degree angle *(left inset)*. Lean forward until your upper body is approximately parallel to the floor, opening the angle of your left knee slightly. Use your free arm to balance *(left)*. Hold for 30-45 seconds. Repeat with your other leg.

Balance and Coordination/5

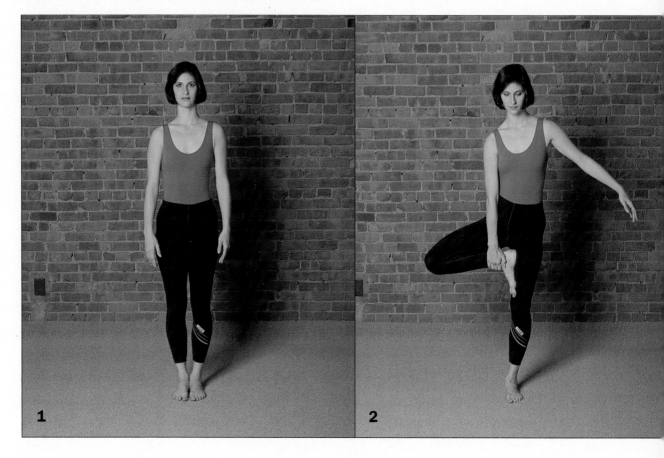

1

2

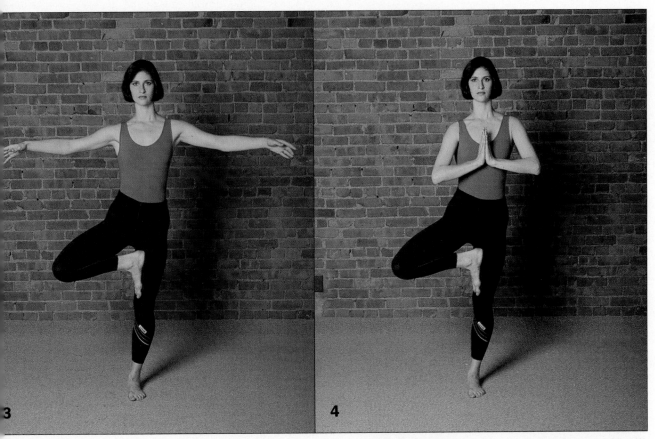

3

4

Stand with your feet together, arms relaxed at your sides (1). With your right hand, grasp the inside of your right ankle and lift your right foot until it rests against the inside of your left thigh (2). Balance in this position for 15 seconds with your arms extended straight out to the sides (3). Bring your hands together at your chest and balance for 30 seconds (4).

Balance and Coordination/6

From a standing position, step forward and bend your right knee in a lunge position while keeping your left leg straight behind you. Raise both arms in front of you at about a 45-degree angle above parallel to the floor *(right inset)*. Bringing your arms downward until they are parallel to the floor, lift your left leg up until it is parallel to the floor *(right)*. Hold for 15 seconds and then repeat with your other leg.

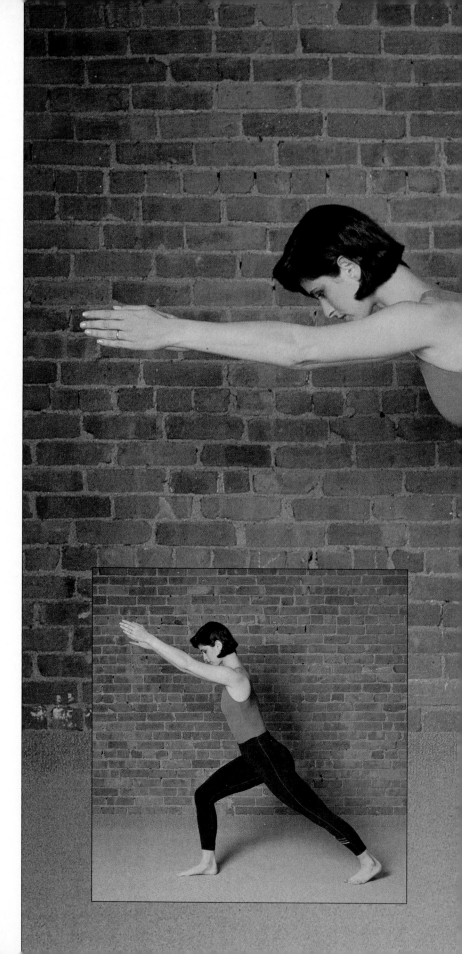

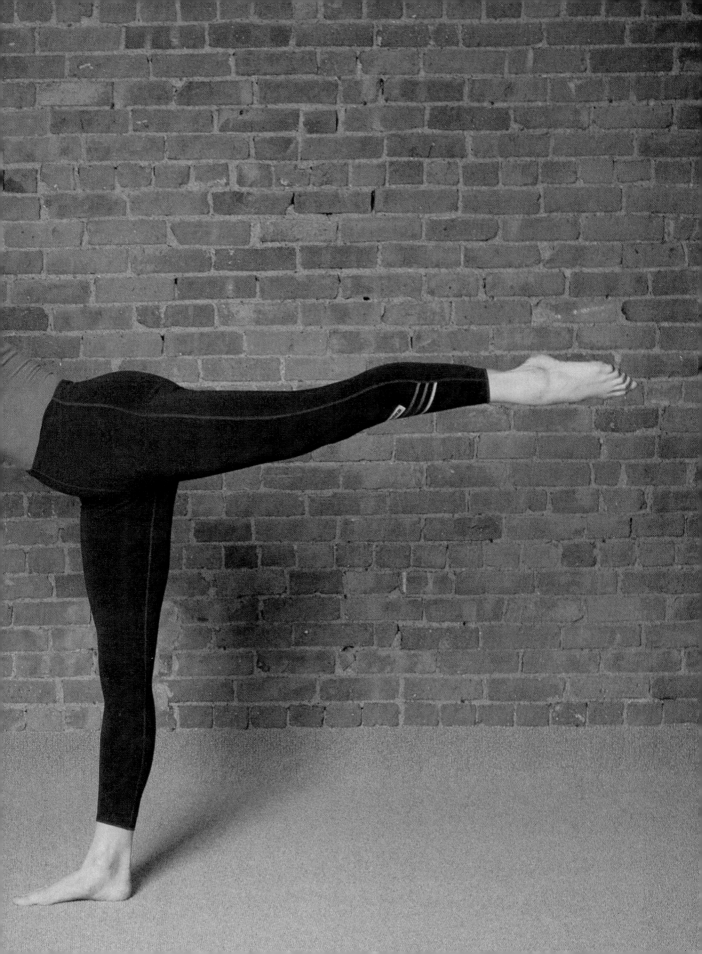

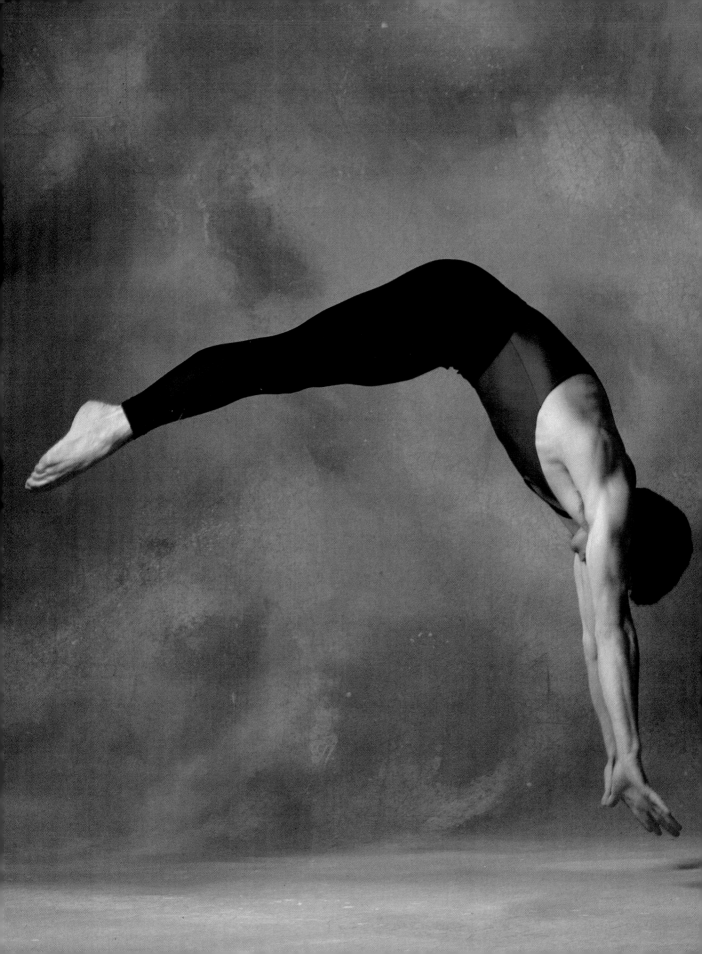

Chapter Three

Tumbling

Gymnastic moves for dexterity and poise

Tumbling involves not only sight and touch but also proprioception — the key inner sense by which you know your orientation in space *(see Chapter Two).* Your senses of sight and touch tell you where your body is in relation to the floor at every stage of a tumbling movement. Proprioception works through sense receptors in the muscles, joints and tendons to assess the force, speed and interrelation of your limbs as you move. In tumbling, this nerve-muscle relationship is combined with the senses of balance and direction, as if the body had a built-in gyroscope to help maintain an overall awareness of position.

A carefully organized program that divides each tumbling skill into its component parts is the basis of safe tumbling, and you can perform the skills demonstrated here with minimal risk. (A few exercises may require the assistance of a spotter, or assistant, depending on your skill level. For tips on spotting, see the box on page 95.) The partner exercises in Chapter Four let you sample a different, though not much more difficult, type of gymnastic movement. If you wish to progress beyond this level (or if you do not currently feel fit enough to begin on your own), join a local club, gym or school with a qualified instructor to pursue your training under professional supervision.

The first exercises in this chapter are movement sequences designed to build conditioning, coordination and flexibility. These are followed by simple tumbling skills, beginning with close-to-the-floor rolls. The forward roll is the basic building block of all tumbling, and variations of it are part of all gymnastics; an aerial somersault on a balance beam or a flying dismount from parallel bars are based on this roll. Practice the rolls until you feel comfortable moving your body through space in these new ways and directions. You will then be ready for variations that require more speed, elevation or prolonged balancing. The stationary balances that follow are also important; handstands and headstands are fundamental to the repertoire. You can learn these balances with the help of a spotter, or by using a wall for support.

A tumbling program requires body strength. A sturdy back and strong arms and legs are crucial, and firm abdominals, besides providing support for movement, work to keep you balanced in stationary poses. Weight training, either with free weights or machines, is a good adjunct to tumbling.

Improving your flexibility is also important. Begin each tumbling session with the exercises described in Chapter Two. They will help prepare you physically and mentally for tumbling. Make sure to perform all parts of the warm-up: Flexible fingers and toes, and well-stretched hip and arm flexors, are valuable assets in tumbling.

The tumbling movements you will learn in this chapter require minimal equipment. You should wear light, comfortable exercise clothes: Sweat pants and shirt, a T-shirt and shorts or a leotard and footless tights are fine. Remove any jewelry, and pull your hair back if it is long, or it may interfere with your vision as you turn or roll. For these exercises, you can be barefoot or wear lightweight sneakers, slip-on dance shoes or gymnastic slippers with suede soles; reinforced running or aerobics shoes are too inflexible and may also throw you off balance.

You will need a large, open space for these exercises. There should be a clear wall space at least five feet wide against which you can practice headstands and backbends. A large, heavyweight exercise mat is the ideal surface for beginners (and is a good investment if you work out at home), but a well-padded carpeted floor is satisfactory at first. Be careful about using a small, lightweight exercise mat; it may slip out from under you as you move. In warm weather, you can also practice outdoors on a level lawn or beach, provided the ground is soft and clear of obstacles.

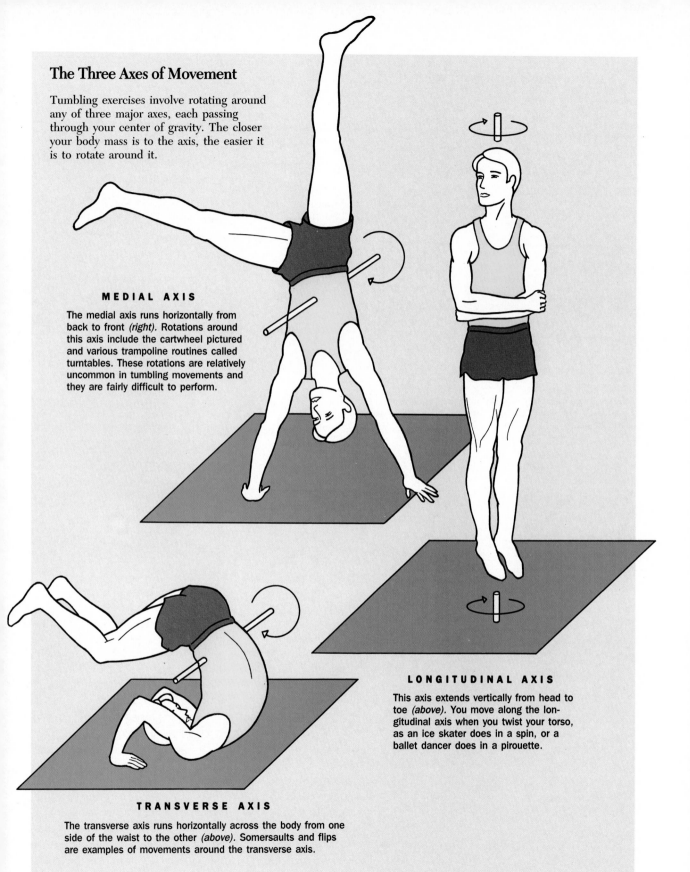

The Three Axes of Movement

Tumbling exercises involve rotating around any of three major axes, each passing through your center of gravity. The closer your body mass is to the axis, the easier it is to rotate around it.

MEDIAL AXIS

The medial axis runs horizontally from back to front *(right)*. Rotations around this axis include the cartwheel pictured and various trampoline routines called turntables. These rotations are relatively uncommon in tumbling movements and they are fairly difficult to perform.

LONGITUDINAL AXIS

This axis extends vertically from head to toe *(above)*. You move along the longitudinal axis when you twist your torso, as an ice skater does in a spin, or a ballet dancer does in a pirouette.

TRANSVERSE AXIS

The transverse axis runs horizontally across the body from one side of the waist to the other *(above)*. Somersaults and flips are examples of movements around the transverse axis.

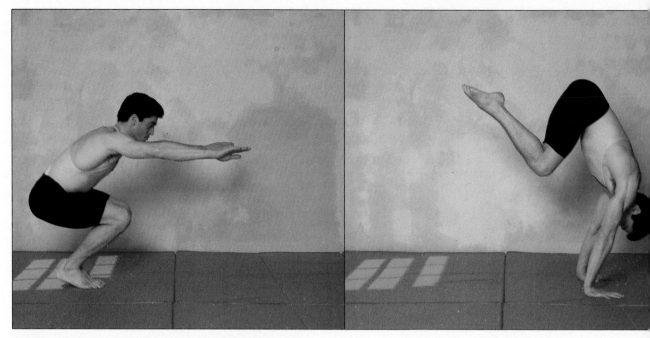

DONKEY KICK Squat down, with your arms extended in front of you. Hop forward, catch your weight on your hands well in front of your body and kick your legs up behind you. Perform eight to 10 repetitions.

Tumbling Conditioners/1

The exercises in this chapter serve three functions: They warm up the body, strengthen arm and leg muscles vital to initiate the momentum required for tumbling movements, and introduce some of the sensations you will encounter in tumbling.

The donkey kick (*above*) uses the calf, thigh and arm muscles, and it familiarizes you with the sensation of supporting your weight on your arms, a posture used repeatedly in tumbling. The front crawl (*above right*) works the biceps; the crab crawl (*right*) develops the triceps.

And both crawl exercises, especially the crab crawl, require coordination: When performing the crab crawl, notice the concentration you need to move your arms and legs for movement in every direction.

The bridge, or backbend, on the following four pages, is an excellent stretch for the back, shoulders and front of the body, and is the basis for advanced gymnastic skills like the back handspring. This position can be a strain for those whose backs are not flexible. If you have lower back problems, you should not attempt to do this exercise.

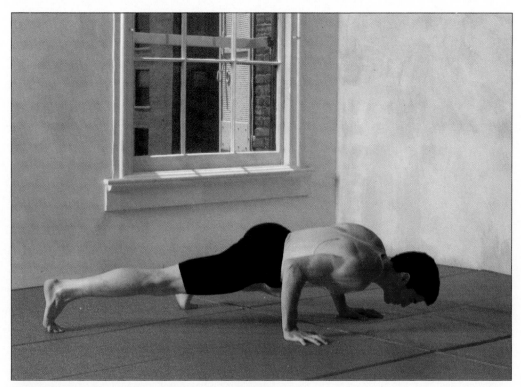

FRONT CRAWL From a push-up position, crawl forward on your hands and toes, staying close to the mat and bringing your knees up close to your body. Keep your torso parallel to the floor as you move.

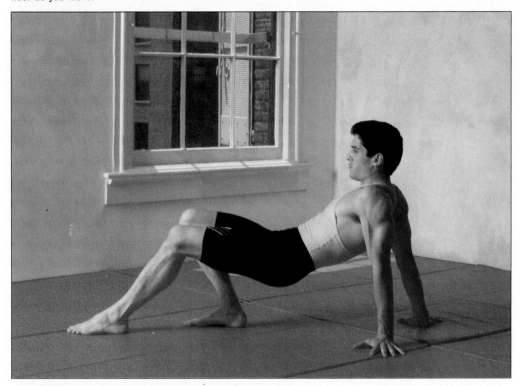

CRAB CRAWL With your arms straight and legs bent, tuck your buttocks beneath you and raise your hips off the mat. Travel forward, backward and sideways, keeping your hips elevated.

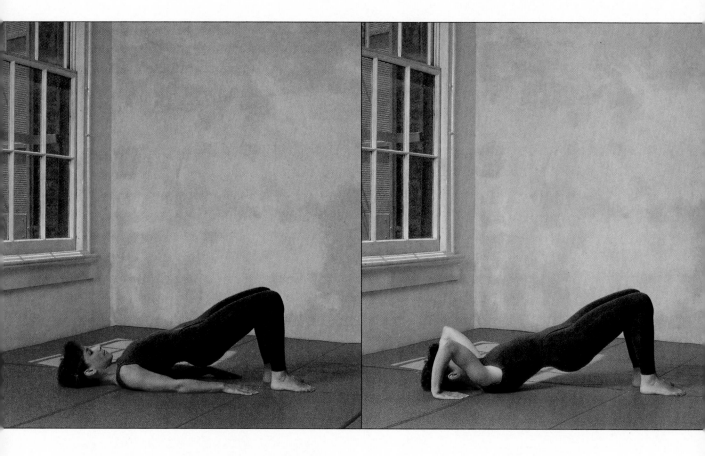

Tumbling Conditioners/2

Lie on the floor with your knees bent, your buttocks tucked and your legs about hip-width apart *(left)*. Place your hands flat on the floor just above your shoulders *(center)*. Lift your body, straightening your arms as much as possible, with your knees bent slightly. Raise your chest high above your arms to form a bridge *(right)*. Hold the position for a few seconds, then drop your hips to the floor. To release your back muscles, hug your knees to your chest and rock back and forth gently.

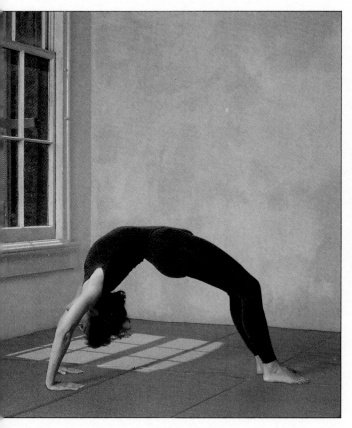

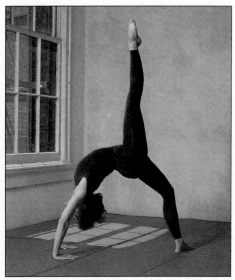

When you feel comfortable holding a bridge, try the following variation: Extend one leg forward, first bent and then straight upward. This position further stretches your back and legs.

Tumbling
Conditioners/3

BACKBEND If you can perform a well-arched bridge on the floor, try to lower yourself to a backbend from a standing position. Stand three feet from a wall, with your feet hip-width apart. Take a deep breath before starting, exhale forcefully as you begin, then breathe normally. Lean backward and place your hands against the wall *(near right)*. Carefully walk your hands down the wall *(center)*. Place your hands flat on the floor and stretch your chest toward the wall *(far right)*. To release your back, lower your hips to the floor and clasp your knees to your chest. If you feel dizzy after holding this position, be sure to allow time for recovery before attempting to stand up.

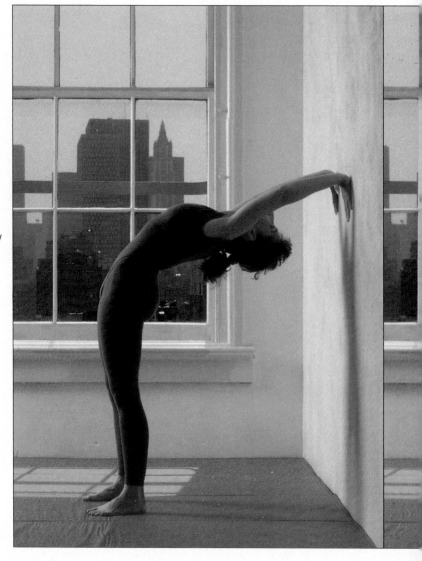

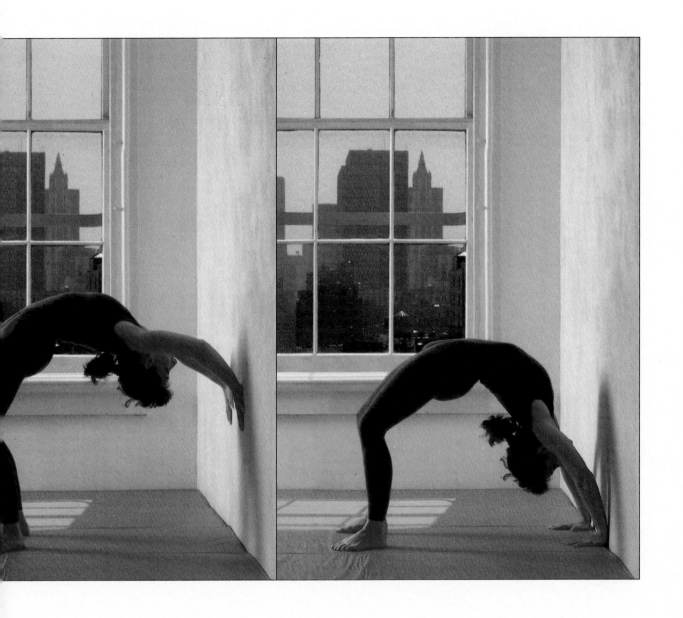

Forward Rolls/1

The forward roll is the basis for many gymnastic skills. The series of rolls on pages 66-71 — the forward roll followed by three variations — is a typical tumbling skill progression. Learn the basic forward roll first, and practice it until you feel comfortable performing it. Always try to roll in a straight line; if you use a mat, stay in the center.

As you roll, bend your body into a curved shape; this tuck position will help you roll smoothly. In order to avoid putting stress on your neck, place your chin on your chest and keep pushing your hands on the floor until your feet come over your head. If you feel dizzy after you finish the roll, stay in a low squat for a few moments before standing up. When you finish a forward roll or any other tumbling skill, hold the final position in your best form for a few seconds.

The one-knee and straddle rolls on pages 68-69 and the dive roll on pages 70-71 require more initial power than the forward roll does because your body forms a less streamlined shape. You must push off with more force from your starting position to propel your body through the whole movement. Start the dive roll by springing off your feet, as you did in the donkey kick.

Start from a squat position, with your arms extended and parallel to the floor (1). Bend forward, place your hands flat on the floor and push off with your toes; let your arms bend to take your weight as you roll forward (2). Tuck your chin as your head, neck and shoulders reach the floor. After you roll, reach forward to bring your weight onto your feet (3). When you regain your balance, stand up (4).

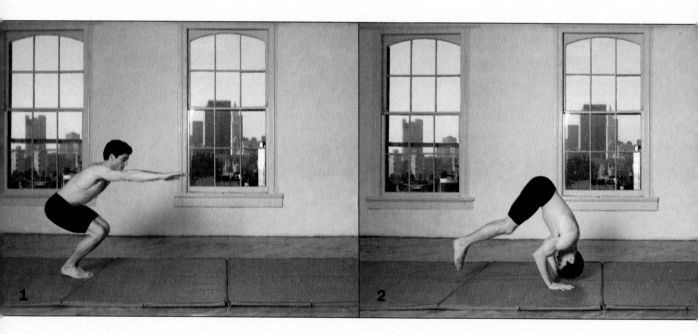

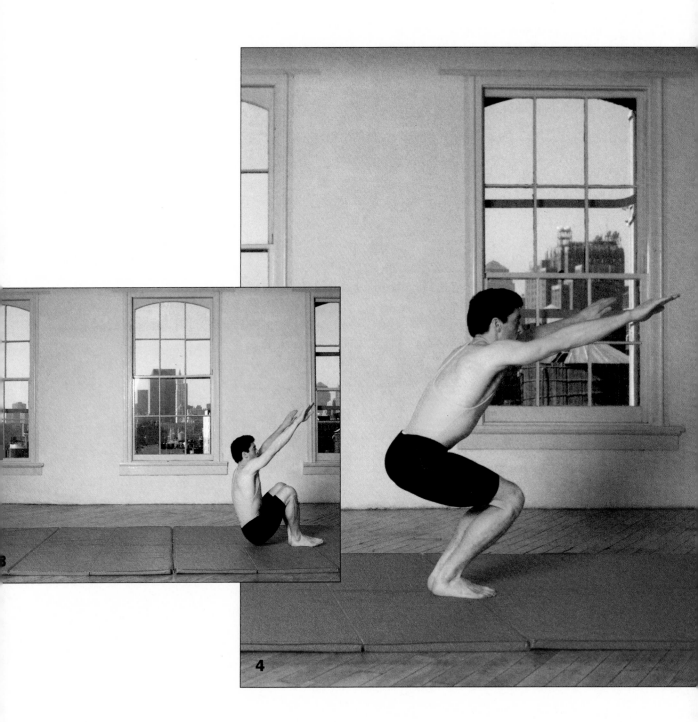

Forward Rolls/2

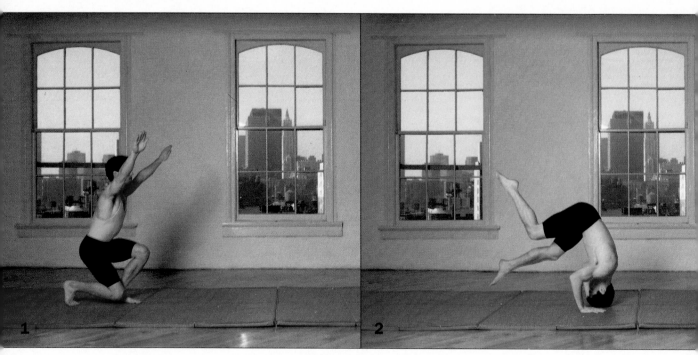

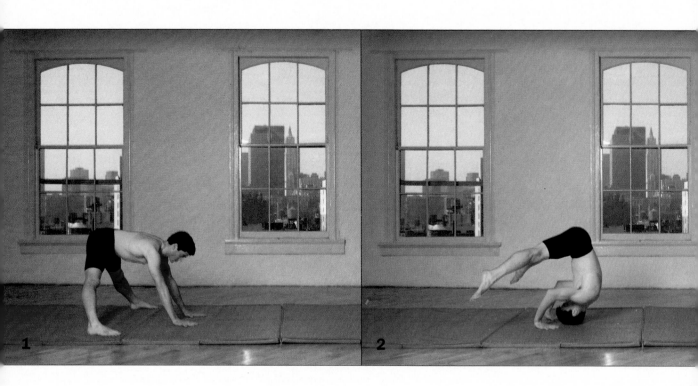

68

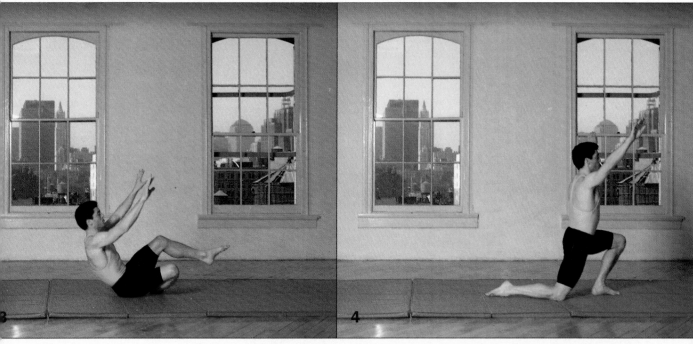

Kneel on your right knee, tuck your toes under, extend your arms upward and push off forcefully with your right foot (1). As you roll, keep your right knee close to your body (2), and come up with your right leg folded under you (3). Place your left foot flat on the mat as you land. Lean forward, raising your arms and arching your back to finish the roll (4).

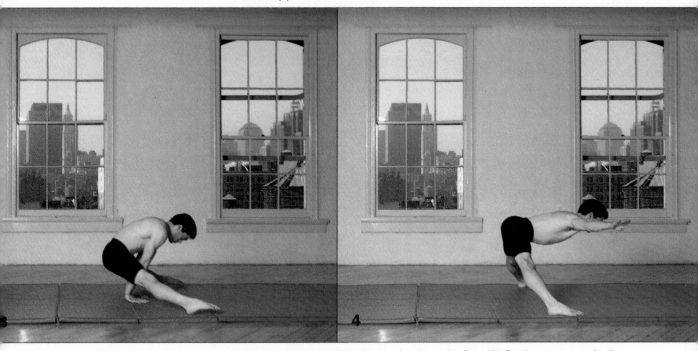

Start in a wide straddle, with your hands on the floor (1). Bend your arms and roll forward forcefully; keep your legs wide apart as they come over your head (2). Pick your hands up and snap them back to the floor in a quick circle, shifting your weight onto your arms (3). Then balance yourself and rise on to your feet, extending your arms to the sides (4).

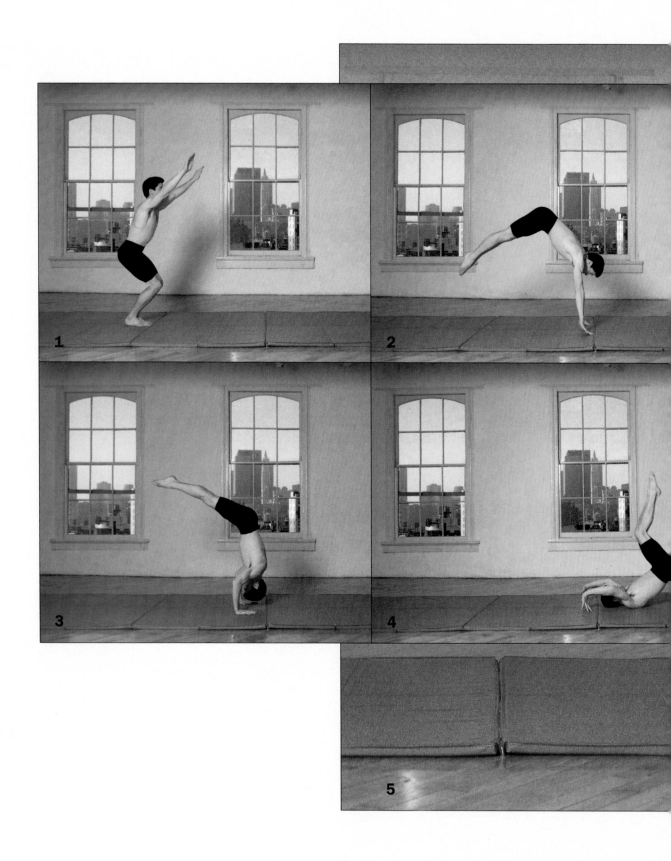

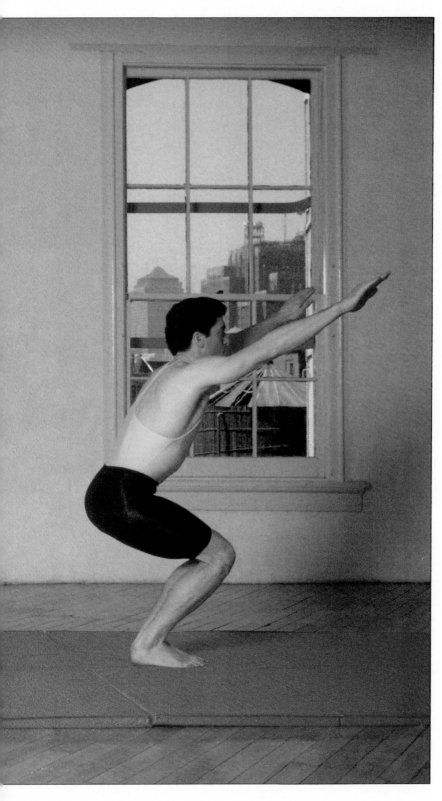

Forward Rolls/3

The dive roll can be performed with a very small hop or with a powerful jump. Begin in a low squat and take just a slight hop to accustom yourself to catching your weight on your hands. As you become more proficient, jump higher and more forcefully, and reach farther forward with your hands as you take off. Stand with your knees bent and arms extended forward and upward (1). Jump with both feet, catching your weight on your hands a short distance in front of your body (2). Bend your arms immediately to absorb the impact (3), tuck your head, round your back and continue the roll (4). Land on your feet, transfer your weight forward and stand up (5).

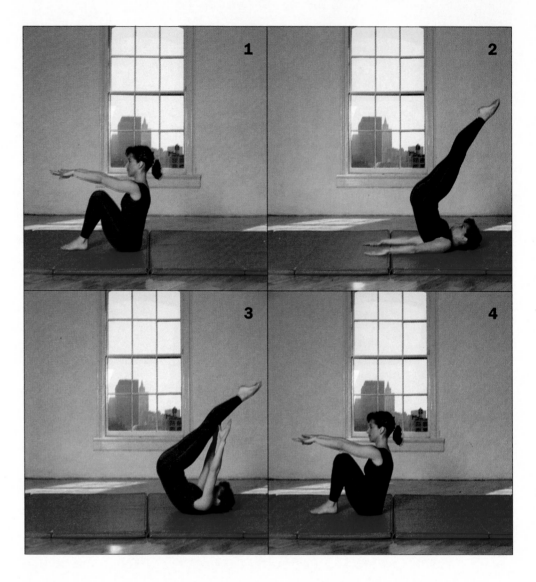

Backward Rolls/1

Although the backward roll appears to be simply the reverse of the forward roll, it is a very different movement and somewhat harder to learn. You may find the sensation of rolling backward unfamiliar and disorienting. Some people have difficulty rolling backward over their heads; be sure to keep it tucked. Place your hands on the floor quickly and use your arms to push your body over, so that your neck and head never support your weight.

The preparatory exercises shown on this page and opposite — the shoulder stand and the half-roll — help you learn the backward roll movement and find the correct spot to place your hands.

When you have mastered the basic backward roll, progress to the first two variations on pages 74-77, in which you begin the roll as usual and then change your leg position to alter the landing. The straddle roll, on pages 78-79, maintains a spread-legged position throughout, and is more difficult; push off forcefully from the start.

Sit with your feet close to your buttocks and arms extended forward (1). Rock backward forcefully, extending your legs. Press your arms against the floor for support and hold the position for a moment (2). Roll back downward and repeat, this time raising your arms toward your knees and balancing for a moment on your upper back and shoulders (3). Roll back to the first position (4).

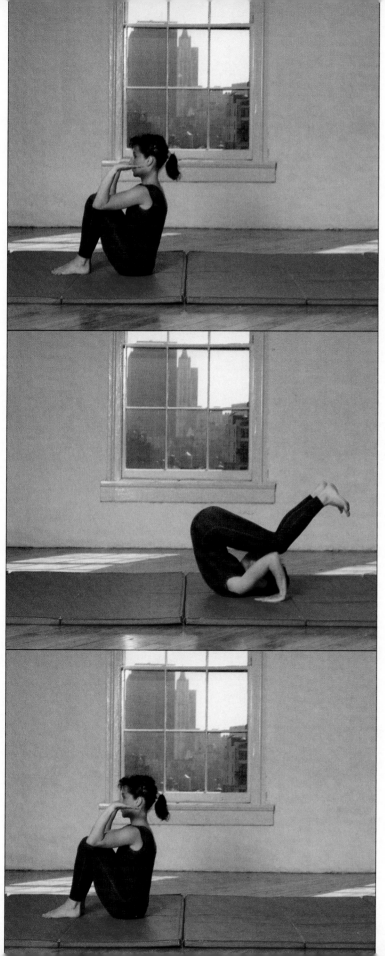

Sit with your feet close to your buttocks and reach your hands back over your shoulders; keep your hands parallel to the floor, with palms up, thumbs toward your ears *(top)*. Roll backward and, before your head touches the floor, place your hands on the floor over your shoulders *(center)*. Catch yourself there and support your weight for a moment, then push off with your hands and roll back to the sitting position *(bottom)*.

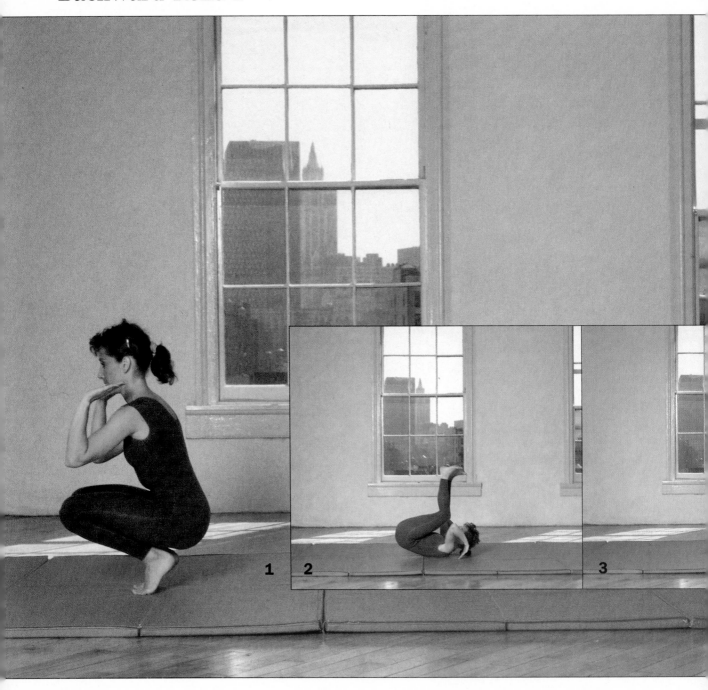

1 2 3

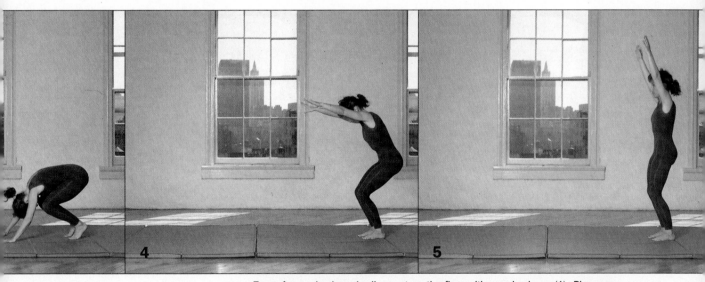

To perform a backward roll, squat on the floor with your heels up (1). Place your hands over your shoulders, parallel to the floor, with your thumbs near your ears. Lean backward until you begin to fall, then push off with your feet to propel your legs over your head. Quickly place your hands on the floor over your shoulders (2). Keep your chin on your chest and push down with your arms as you roll over your neck and head. Land on your feet in a squat (3), and begin to rise. Pause briefly in a partial squat until you regain your balance (4). Stand with arms extended to finish (5).

Backward Rolls/3

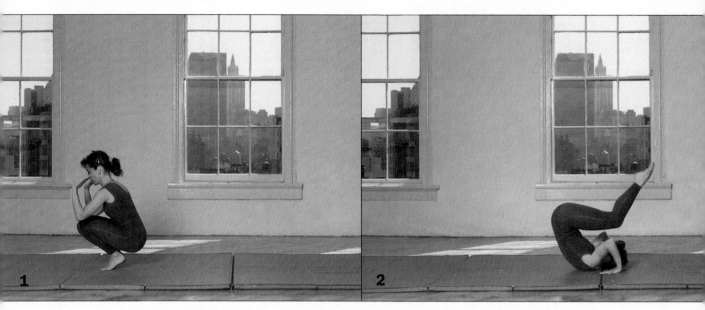

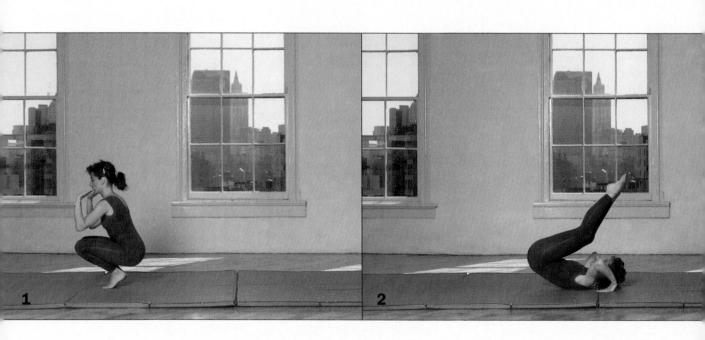

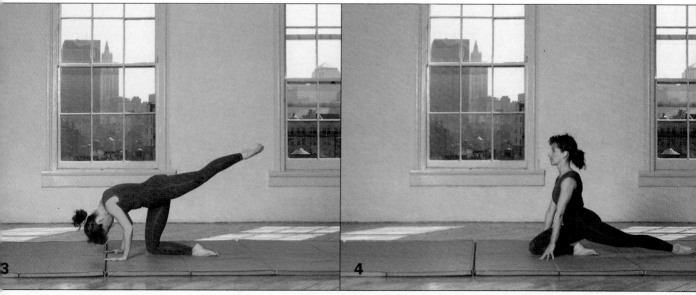

This roll requires more momentum, as the extended leg interrupts the smooth, rolling motion. Begin a basic backward roll (1). Keep your knees close to your chest as your feet come over your head (2). Land on your right knee and extend your left leg (3). Lower your left leg to the floor, sit on your right heel and push your upper body upward with your arms (4).

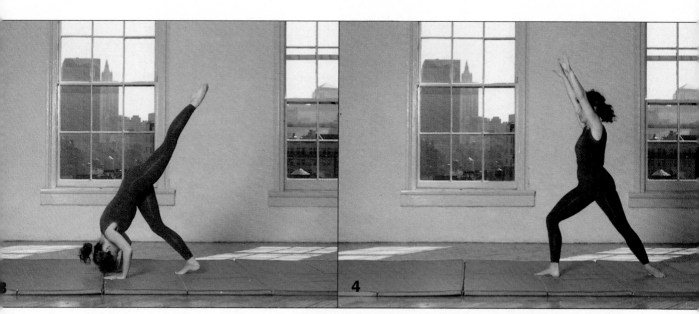

Begin a basic backward roll (1, 2). As your legs come toward the floor, keep your arms bent, bring your right knee close to your chest and flex your right foot so that you land on it, then straighten your leg (3). Push off forcefully with your arms to raise your body and continue to reach upward as you simultaneously lower your left leg (4).

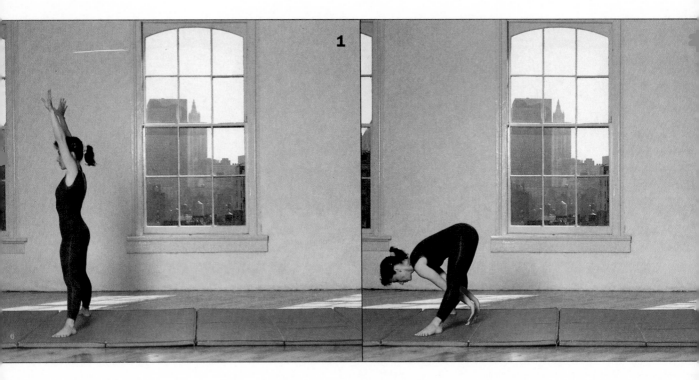

1

Backward Rolls/4

The straddle backward roll requires powerful arms and a quick movement. Stand in a wide straddle, with your feet parallel and arms extended above your head (1). Keep your legs straight as you lean your upper body forward and begin to sit down. Reach between your legs and place your hands, fingers facing forward, on the floor to catch your weight (2). When your buttocks touch the floor (3), reach your arms overhead and push over in a regular backward roll; keep your legs apart (4). As your toes reach the floor, push up forcefully with your hands to bring your chest parallel to the floor (5). Extend your arms to the sides, arch your back slightly and hold the position for a moment (6).

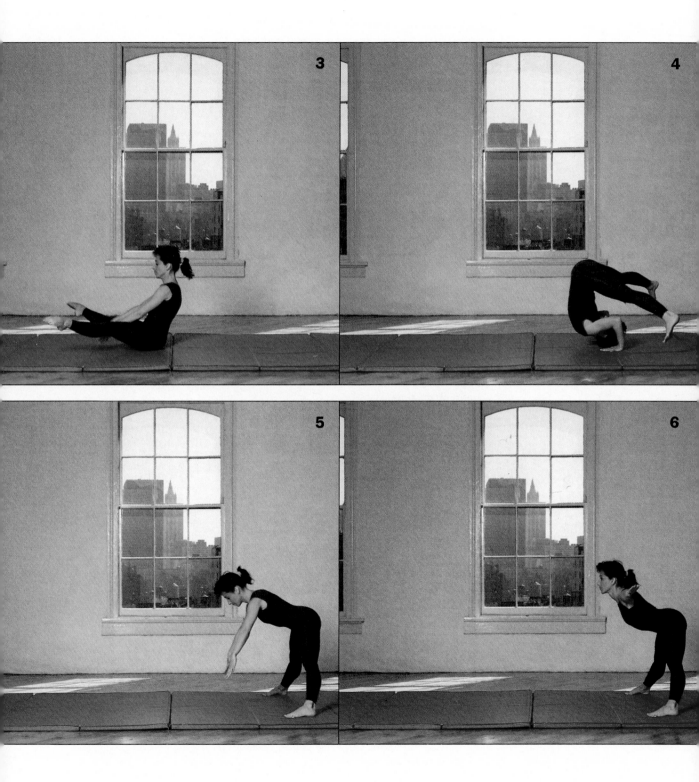

Balancing/1

This sequence of skills will help you develop the balance and body control necessary to hold a headstand or handstand. Strong arms are an asset, but your abdominal muscles — your center — will support you in these positions. You can begin by picking up either your left or right foot first; alternate so you feel comfortable leading with either one.

Concentration is also important in holding a balance. When you are comfortable in a headstand, you will find the position restful and refreshing. However, your first headstand can be disconcerting; the blood rushes to your head and your heart pounds. Take plenty of time to regain your balance before standing up; kneel with your head down for a few minutes if you continue to feel dizzy, and get up slowly.

The two preparatory exercises on this page can be performed alone; for the headstand and handstand, you should enlist someone as a spotter. If possible, take turns spotting so that each of you can experience both activities.

The spotter should focus on the performer's hips. Once they are positioned over the shoulders, the spotter can help align the performer's legs. The spotter should not force the legs into place, but should catch and hold them lightly until the performer finds his own balance.

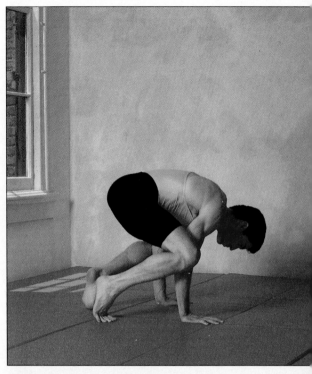

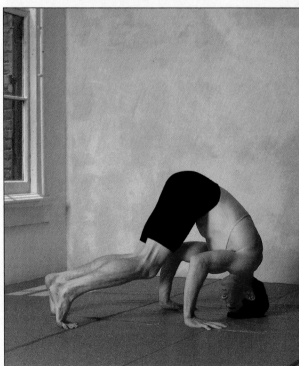

Place your hands on the mat shoulder-width apart. Place your forehead on the mat about one foot in front of your hands *(above)*. Bring your knees up to rest on your elbows and balance for a few moments *(center)*. This balance is called a tripod *(right)*.

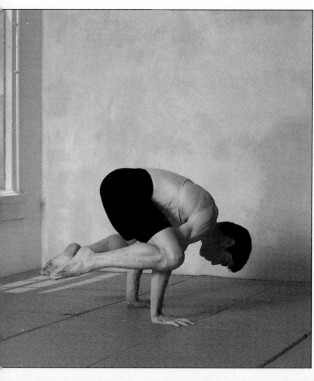

Squat with your hands shoulder-width apart on the mat.
Press your knees against the outsides of your elbows
(far left), rock forward to bring your feet up, so that
your lower legs are parallel to the floor, and hold for a
moment *(left)*.

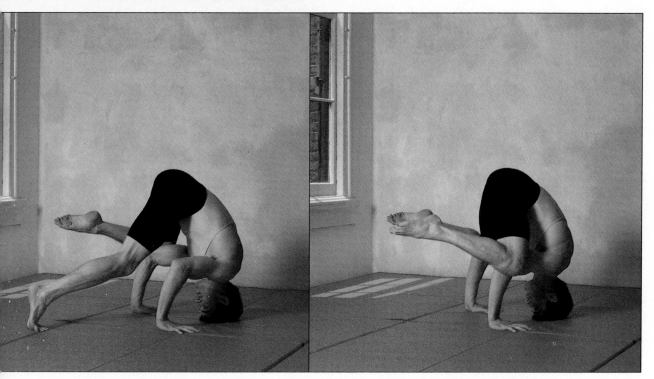

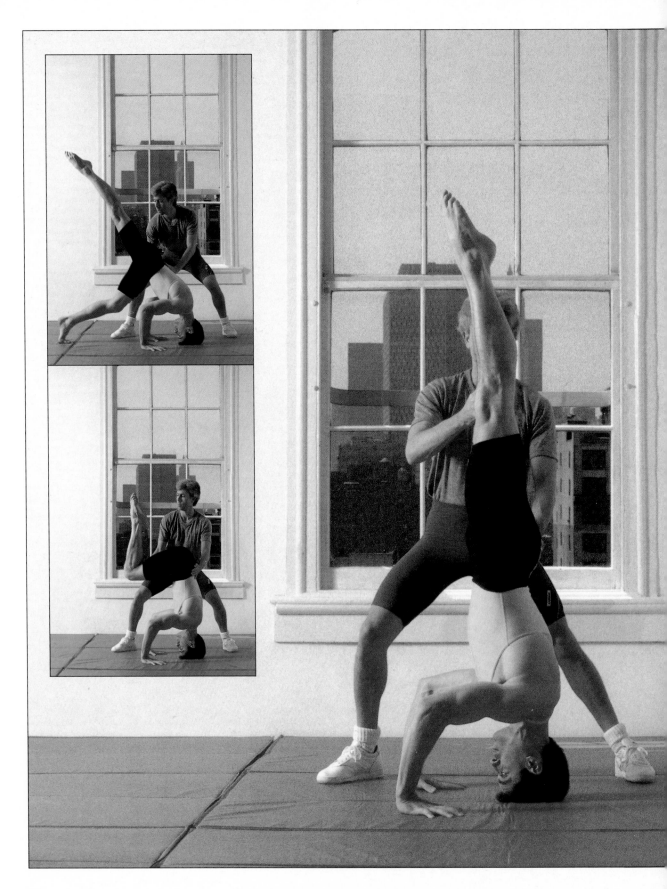

Balancing/2

HEADSTAND Have a spotter stand at your left side before you begin. Place your hands and head on the floor as you did for the tripod. The spotter places his left hand on your lower back. Straighten your left leg and raise it as high as you can *(far left, top).* As you raise your right knee, bend your left knee and bring your legs together *(far left, bottom).* The spotter supports your left thigh with his right hand. Slowly raise your legs straight upward. The spotter guides your legs and holds them lightly at the knees *(near left).* If you are able to balance, he can let go, but should keep his hands close to your knees. Tighten your buttocks and abdominal muscles and point your toes; breathe normally. Lower one leg at a time and rest in a kneeling position for a moment before standing up.

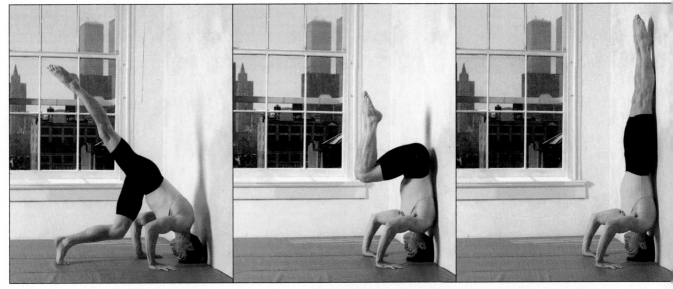

Place your head close to the wall and your hands on the floor shoulder-width apart about a foot in front of the wall. Raise your left leg *(left).* As you lift your right knee up, bend your left knee and bring your legs together; your back should be touching the wall *(center).* Stay in this position or slowly straighten both legs and let them rest against the wall *(right).* Lower your legs one at a time and kneel, head down, until you regain your balance.

Balancing/3

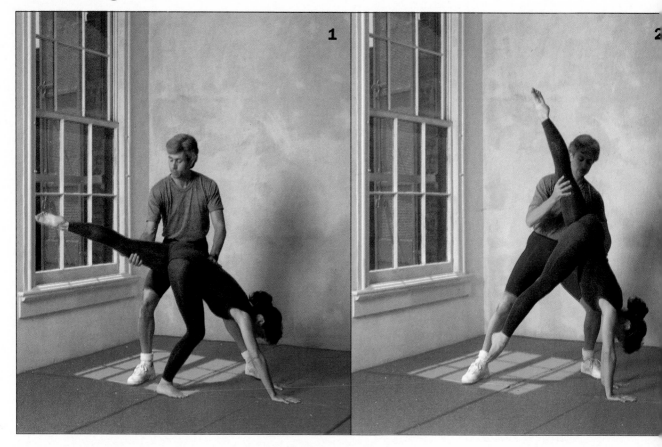

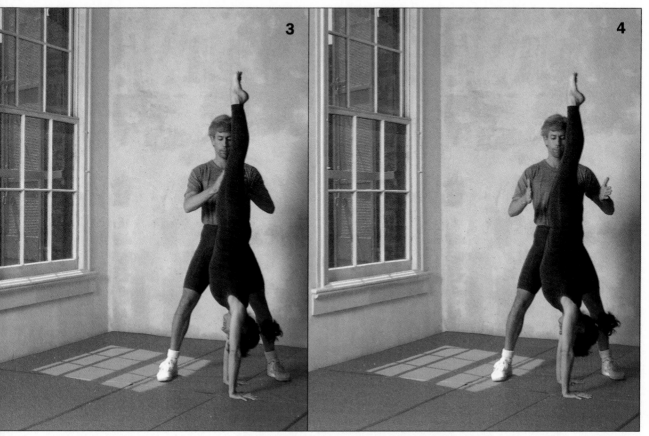

HANDSTAND The spotter should stand at your left side before you begin. Place your hands shoulder-width apart on the floor, about three feet in front of your feet. Spread your fingers slightly and arch your palms. Keep your head between your arms throughout the exercise, focusing your eyes on the floor. Raise your left leg as high as you can. The spotter places his left hand on your lower back and supports your left thigh with his right hand (1). Push off with your right foot and continue to lift your left leg. The spotter, still supporting your back, helps you lift your leg (2). Bring your right leg up to meet your left, perpendicular to the floor. Keep your buttocks tucked, your abdominal muscles tight and your toes pointed (3). If you can balance, the spotter may remove his hands, but should keep them close to your legs, ready to assist you (4). Lower one leg at a time with the spotter's assistance, and stand up slowly.

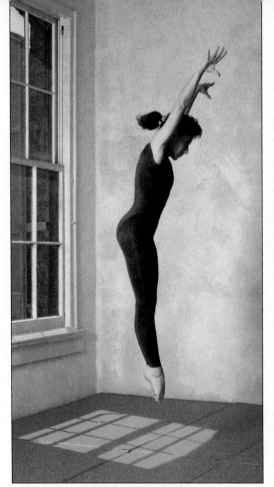

STRAIGHT JUMP With your arms at your sides, jump up, swinging your arms forward and above your head. Land securely with your knees bent.

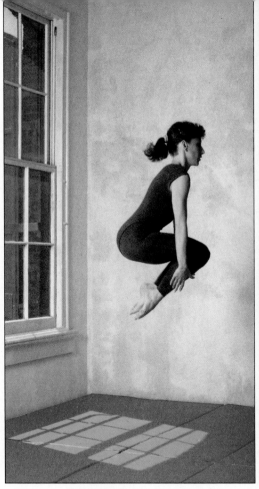

TUCK JUMP Sweep your arms upward, then swing them downward again, as you jump up quickly and tuck your knees into your chest.

In the Air/1

The cartwheel and roundoff, shown on pages 88-91, are the most advanced tumbling skills in this book. Both begin with skip steps, used in tumbling as takeoffs and transitions: A skip and jump transforms forward speed into upward thrust. The jumps shown here build leg strength, providing the power needed for tumbling quickly. These jumps require body control and coordination; try to do them in good form, keeping your abdominal muscles tight and your toes pointed.

Do a small cartwheel at first, barely lifting your feet from the floor. Gradually kick higher until your legs travel over your head during the movement. In a roundoff, the leg and hand positions change slightly, leading to a landing different from the cartwheel finish. The roundoff is often used to build momentum for such skills as back handsprings; it is usually performed with such great force that the gymnast rebounds high into the air at the finish. Start slowly, building power as you master the skill.

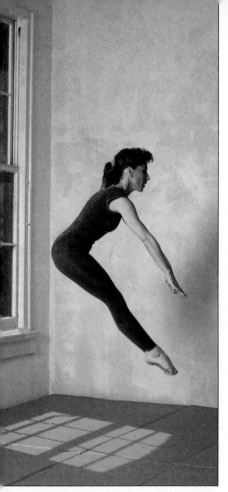

PIKE JUMP Start with your arms over your head, then swing them downward in front of you as you jump and swing your legs forward forcefully.

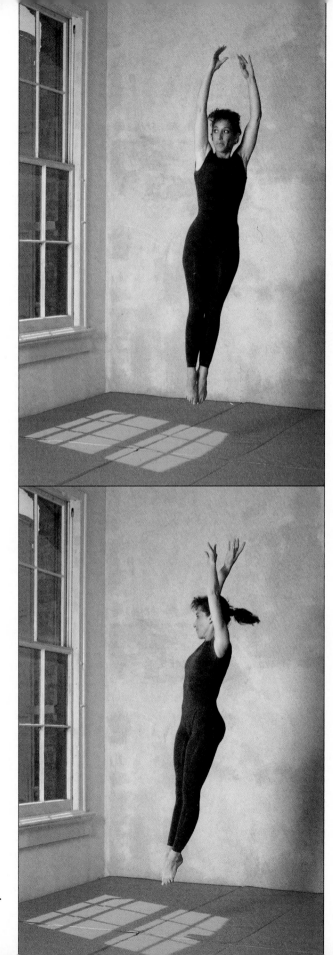

JUMP-TURN Start with your arms at your sides, then sweep them upward as you jump and turn. Turn halfway around (180 degrees) at first, then try for a full turn (360 degrees), landing on the same spot.

In the Air/2

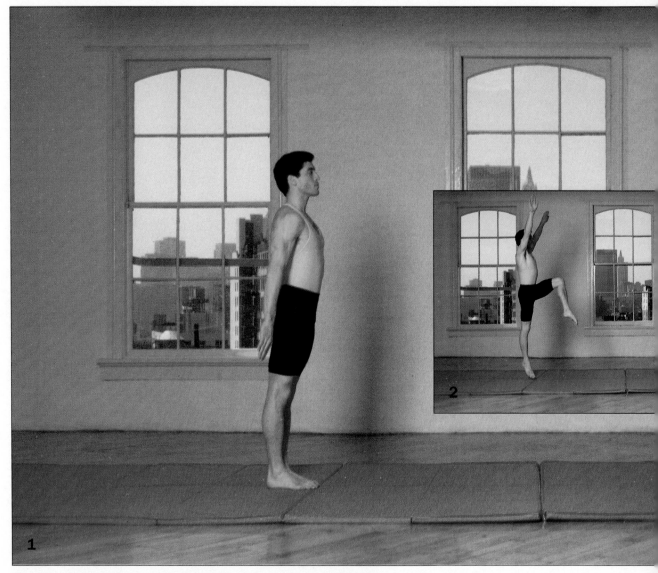

1

2

Begin the cartwheel with a short skip-step in place. Keep your eyes on the floor, following an imaginary straight line. Stand straight, with your arms at your sides (1). Swing your arms upward as you take a skip-step on your right foot, lifting your left knee (2). As your left foot touches the floor, bend your knee and lunge off this leg, straightening it as you do. Place your left hand, fingers pointing left, on the floor (3), and kick your right leg over your head. Place your right hand two to three feet from your left hand; land on your left foot (4) and, as your right foot lands, push your body up to a standing position (5).

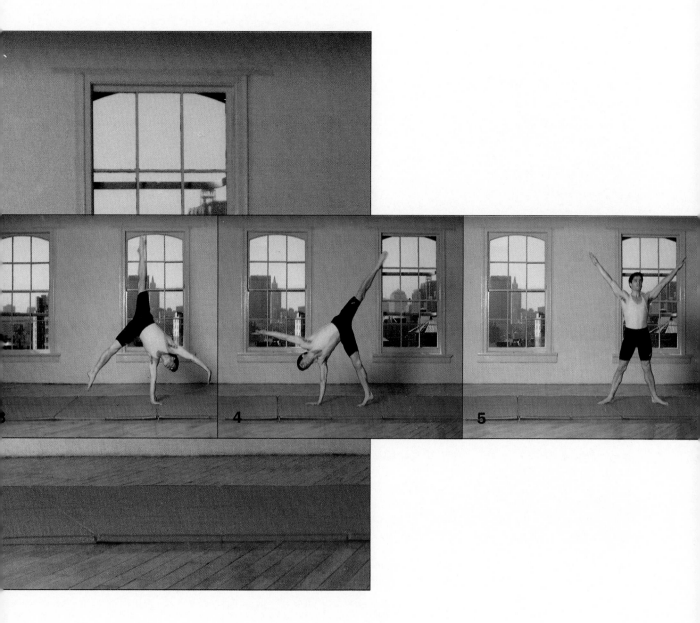

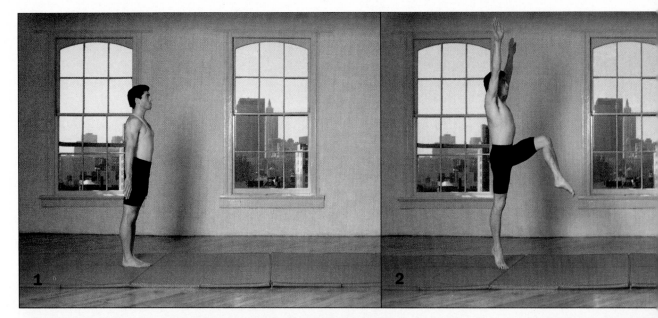

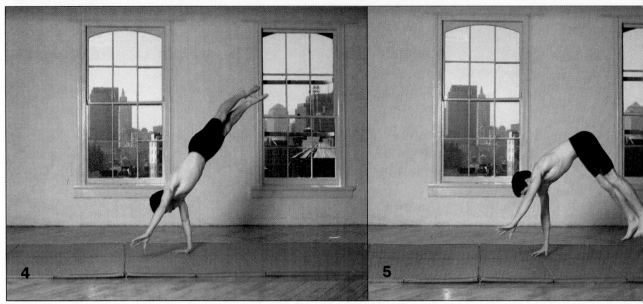

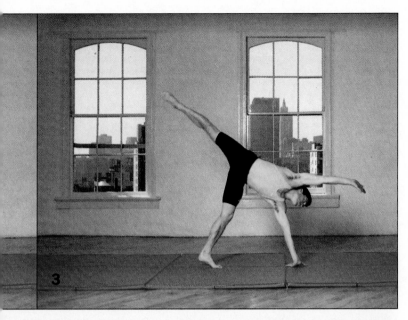

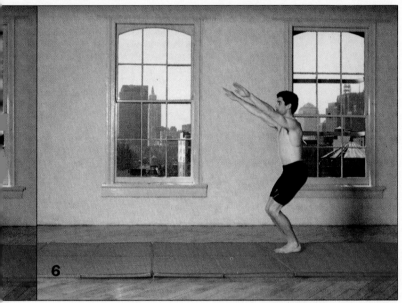

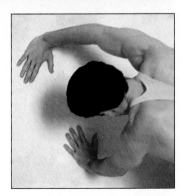

In the Air/3

In a roundoff, place your right hand beyond your left to turn your body sideways. The picture at left shows the right hand landing as the body begins to turn. Begin a cartwheel (1-3), but place your right hand on the floor beyond your left hand, fingers pointing inward. Bring your left leg up to meet your right leg, pivoting your body to the right (4). Push off your hands forcefully and snap both legs down together (5) as you raise your upper body. Land with your knees bent (6).

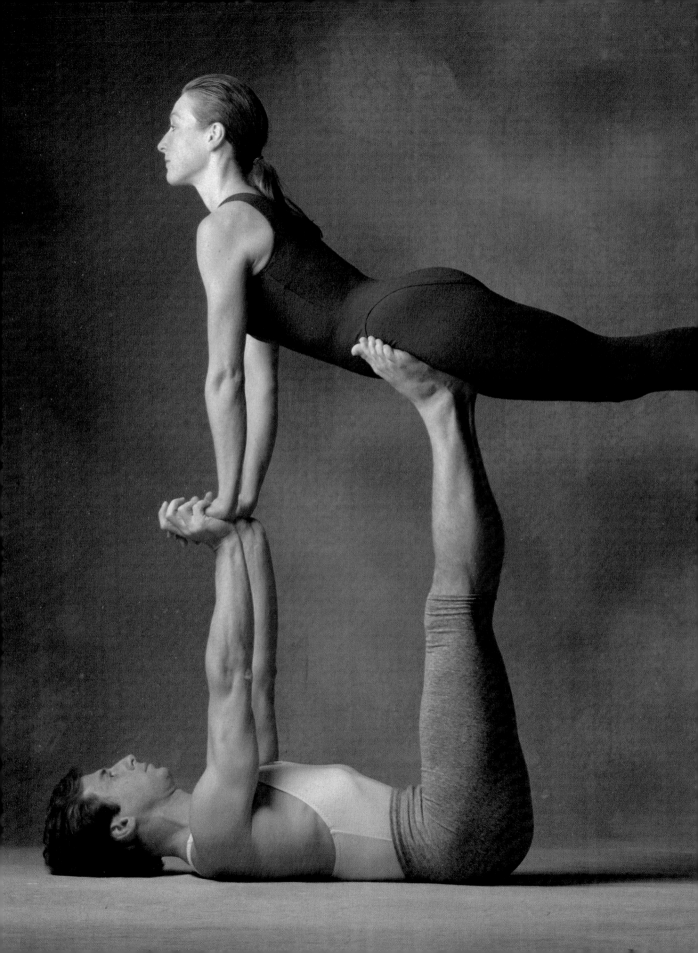

CHAPTER FOUR

Partner Exercise

Agility through synchronicity

A s any ballroom dancer knows, synchronizing one's movement with the steps and motions of a partner is harder to do than it looks. The dynamic activity of dance and gymnastics tends to accentuate differences between bodies, so partners must adapt their movements to compensate for the dissimilarities. And they must do so without looking unbalanced or awkward since form is of paramount importance whether it applies to a tumbling routine or dancing. Working with a partner on the gymnastic exercises in this chapter will help you develop your ability to move gracefully together in addition to refining your sense of balance and building your strength.

Movement exercises with another person require cooperation and sensitivity to the ways in which your individual physical characteristics and abilities blend with your partner's. He or she may not only be different from you in height and size, but stronger or more flexible in certain areas of the body, weaker and less pliable in others. One of you may not balance as easily as the other. Each of these differences will influence how you perform as a team.

Exercising with a partner while minimizing your differences adds another dimension to body awareness that you will not experience if you exercise by yourself. Moving in synchronized fashion, balancing your bodies in unusual positions and helping each other to stretch a little farther and in ways that would be impossible on your own will not only increase your knowledge of how your body performs gymnastic moves but will also provide clues about your posture and movement during everyday activities. These insights will enable you to improve your grace and coordination when you are without your partner as well as when you interact as a duo.

In addition to increasing your body awareness, the exercises in this chapter will help you learn to balance with a partner. Balance of any kind is a dynamic activity, not a static one. At all times, whether you are aware of it or not, you are in constant motion. Even when you are not exercising or consciously moving about, you are never entirely still. If you simply stand next to your partner and pay attention to each other and yourself, you will see that your bodies are really anything but motionless. You are engaged in a rotational dance of breathing and subtle muscle movements that maintain your posture.

Similarly, when you balance as a couple, you actually move and readjust your body position in a much more complex way, as opposed to when you move individually, since you must take into account the forces you both exert on each other as well. This makes a pose held by two people more difficult to maintain than a pose by one person.

While you develop your ability to balance with a partner as you work through the exercises and poses in this chapter — especially when you balance on all fours or on your stomach — you will strengthen muscles that your body uses to stabilize its posture in various positions. These muscles may not be developed adequately during ordinary daily movement. For example, when you balance across your partner during the exercise on page 116, your support comes from your abdominal and back muscles. In contrast, when you stand with one leg off the floor, as instructed on page 112, you use and develop extra strength in the quadriceps, the thigh muscles in the front of the supporting leg. You perform a strengthening exercise that flexes the muscles of your raised leg as you hold the position.

These exercises are based on strength-building calisthenics and weight-training routines like the squat and the push-up, but they use the body weight of your partner instead of your own weight or that of a barbell to develop your muscle strength. Because you can vary the amount of resistance by placing your partner in various positions, you can suit the level of difficulty to your own capabilities. As your strength grows, you can make the exercises more taxing.

Balancing on one leg, as the exercise on pages 114-115 requires, also challenges and fine-tunes your balancing ability. When you stand on both feet and your center of gravity oscillates, you can remain

Working with a Partner

Spotting means helping exercisers perform movements while watching for incorrect body positions that could lead to injuries. Spotting takes practice. You should never try a very difficult gymnastic routine without being spotted by someone who knows how to react to keep you safe if you make a mistake. In some exercises, a partner acts as a spotter. When spotting or being spotted, keep the following points in mind:

◆ Both the exerciser and the spotter should have a good knowledge of the activity to be performed. The exerciser, in particular, should have practiced and mastered the basic component skills that go into the movement.

◆ The spotter should be extremely attentive to the exerciser's movement and should not let his or her attention wander at any time during the exercise. Use two spotters if there is any doubt about one spotter's ability to supervise the exercise safely.

◆ In most cases, the spotter should focus attention on the exerciser's center of gravity, the area around the hips. When supporting or coaching the exerciser through a gymnastic movement, apply force at this area. Often, pressure applied to this part of the body is safest and most effective for helping someone complete an exercise.

upright as long as your center stays over the area bordered by your feet. On one leg, however, unless you keep your center of gravity over the much smaller area that is directly under your supporting foot, you will lose your balance and fall. Because you are never entirely still, this can be difficult.

Performing this exercise and the other movements and poses in this chapter also demonstrates the unique aspect of gymnastics and dance that many other fitness activities lack — the creation of graceful motions that are pleasing to the eye. While elegant movement may be a by-product of other kinds of exercise and athletic performance, it is a central goal of gymnastics and dance.

The exercises shown on pages 96-99 are warm-up stretches that should be performed before moving on to the other activities. The last three exercises, shown on pages 118-123, are significantly more difficult than the exercises in the rest of the chapter and should only be attempted if you are proficient in performing handstands, if you have mastered the rest of the chapter and if you are free of back problems or other limiting physical conditions. If you have back trouble, avoid exercises such as the ones on pages 107, 118-119 and 120-121, which require you to arch your back. That kind of motion can aggravate back problems. Always use caution with all of these exercises, and refrain from completing any movement that begins to cause pain or discomfort.

Partner Stretching/1

Development and mainte-nance of flexibility is prob-ably the most neglected area of fitness for a simple reason — most people find it boring to stretch. However, stretching is a vital component of any fitness program. The flexibility you develop will increase (or at least maintain) the range of motion of your joints and, consequently, it will enhance your ability to perform many activities.

Performing stretches with a part-ner offers a wider selection of activi-ties than when you stretch alone. The extra support and push you get from a partner also allows you to stretch farther than you can during solo stretches.

The stretches shown here and on pages 98-99 allow you to push and pull against your partner. As you do these exercises, allow the motions to create a substantial feeling of stretching in the involved muscles, but be careful not to push yourselves too hard. Hold each stretch for 15-30 seconds. Be sure to breathe normally during each stretch.

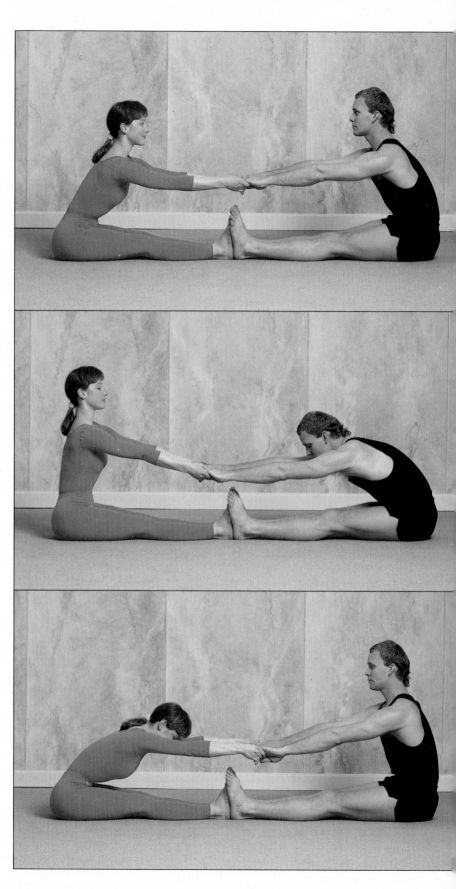

Sit with your feet straight in front of you, heel to heel with your partner, and hold your partner's hands. Keep your knees straight *(top)*. **SHE:** Gently pull backward while your partner leans forward as much as possible. Hold the position *(center)*. Then lean in the opposite direction and hold *(bottom)*.

Sit back to back, with your knees bent, feet either flat on the floor or with your legs crossed *(top right)*. **SHE:** Lean for-ward as far as possible, with your arms extended over your head. **HE:** Lean back-ward, letting your weight press down against her, with your arms extended *(center right)*. After holding the position, lean in the opposite direction and hold *(bottom right)*.

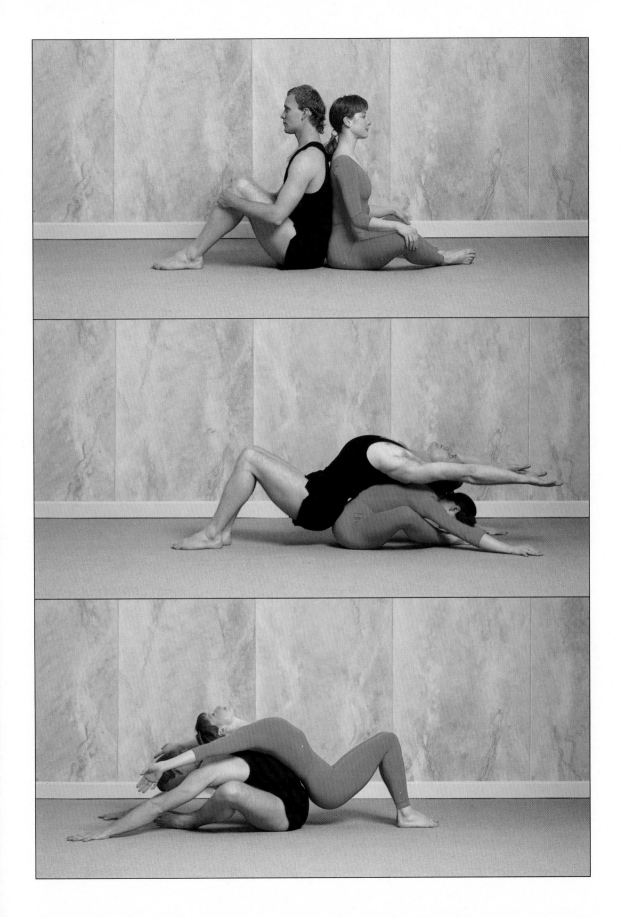

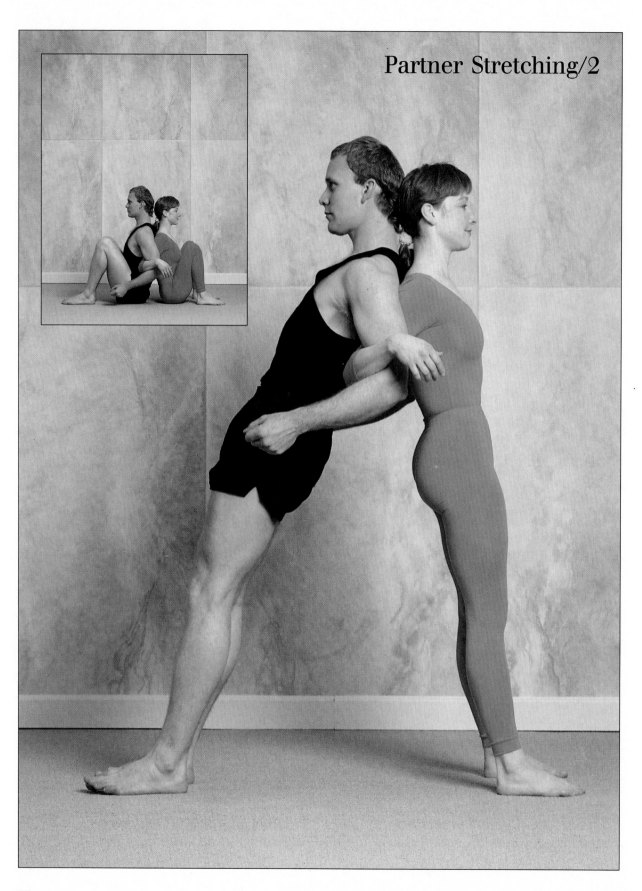

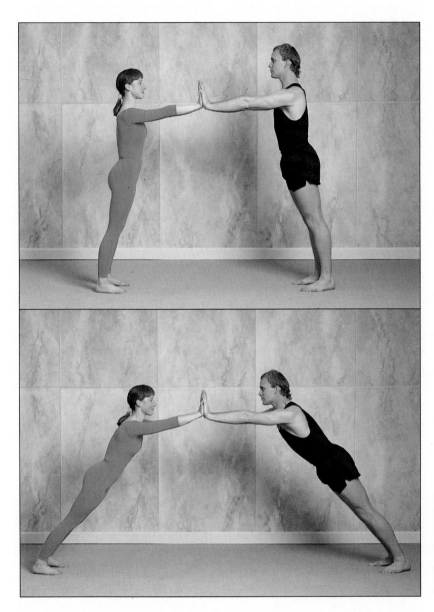

Stand about five feet in front of your partner and extend your arms forward, palm to palm with your partner *(above left).* While leaning forward, both partners slowly step backward while still pressing palms together until your bodies are at approximately a 60-degree angle with the floor *(left).* Hold this position. Walk toward each other to stand up straight.

Sit back to back with your knees bent, feet flat on the floor and arms interlocked with your partner *(inset).* Without unlocking your arms, stand up slowly, paying special attention to keep your balance *(left).* Hold this position.

Routines for Strength/1

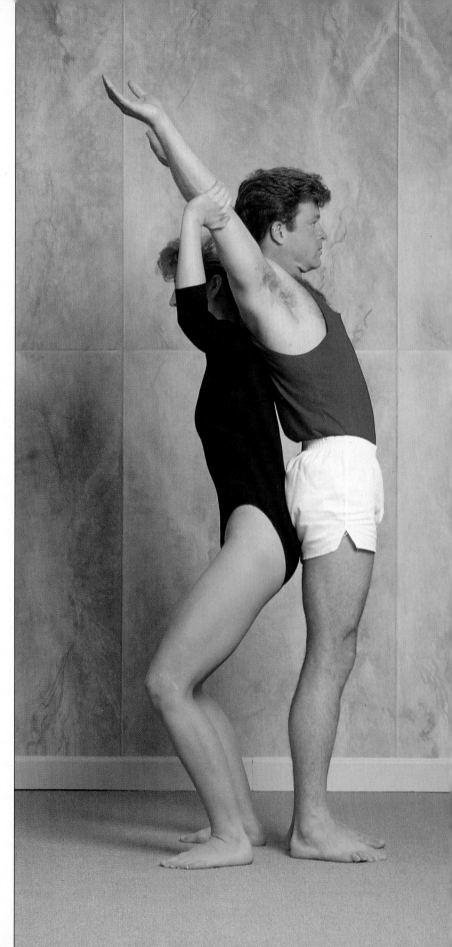

The strength-developing exercises on these two pages and on pages 102-105 are all derived from standard calisthenic and strength-building movements. In each one, your partner's body increases the difficulty of the exercise either by requiring you to support his or her weight, or by increasing the distance through which you have to lower and raise your own body weight.

The exercise shown on these two pages is a variation of a standard squat. However, unlike the usual squat, which is performed with a barbell held across your shoulders, this squat distributes your partner's weight well across your back.

The exercises on pages 102-105 are variations on push-ups and hip dips. By elevating your feet, these exercises increase the development of your arms and shoulders.

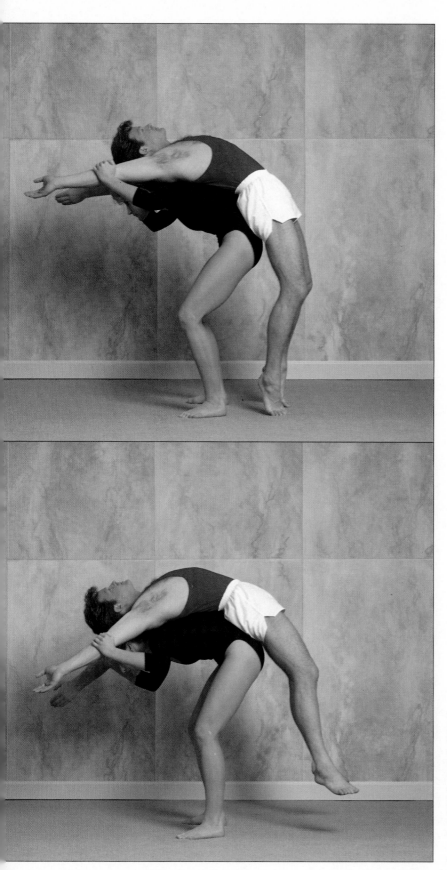

Stand back to back with your partner.
HE: Lift your arms straight over your head
and lean backward. **SHE:** Bend your knees
and grasp his arms at the elbows *(far left)*.
SHE: Lean forward, pulling him up and
onto your back. **HE:** Come up on your toes
as you lean backward *(top left)*. **SHE:** Continue to lean forward until your back is
almost parallel with the floor. **HE:** Allow your
feet to come off the floor with your
weight entirely supported by your partner
(bottom left). Hold this position for 10
seconds. Switch positions and repeat.

101

Routines for Strength/2

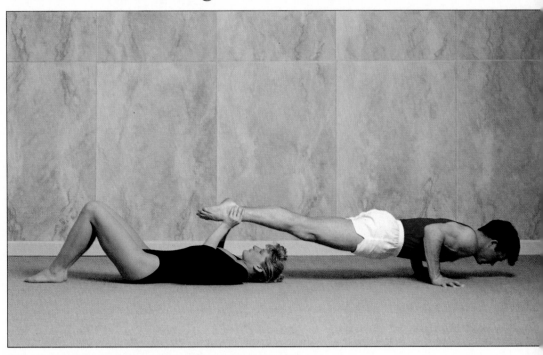

SHE: Lie on your back with your knees bent and feet flat on the floor, and with your arms bent, grasp his ankles. **HE:** Assume the push-up position with your arms bent and chest six inches above the floor *(above left)*. **SHE:** Straighten your arms and lift his feet as high as possible. **HE:** Push up and straighten your arms *(above right)*. Do five repetitions. Switch positions and repeat.

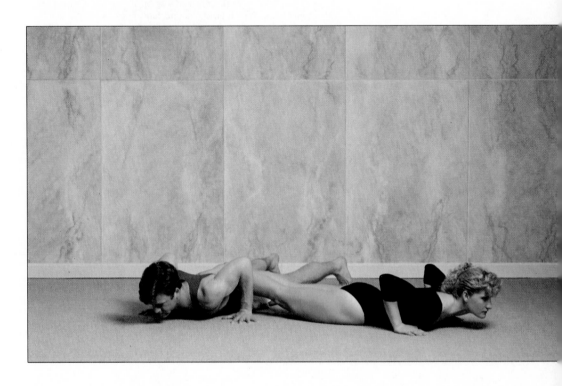

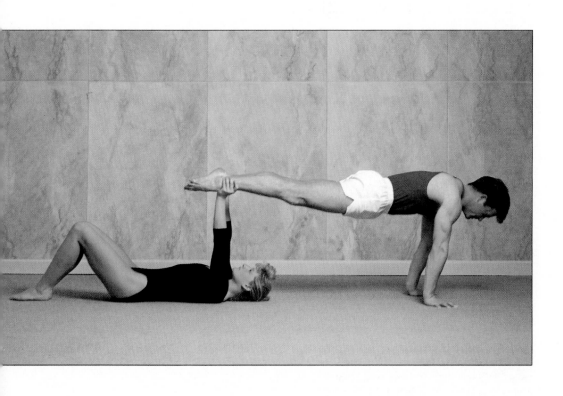

Both partners assume the push-up position with arms bent and chest on the floor. **SHE:** Lie at a right angle to him with your shins on his back *(below left).* Both partners push up *(below right).* Do five repetitions. Switch positions and repeat.

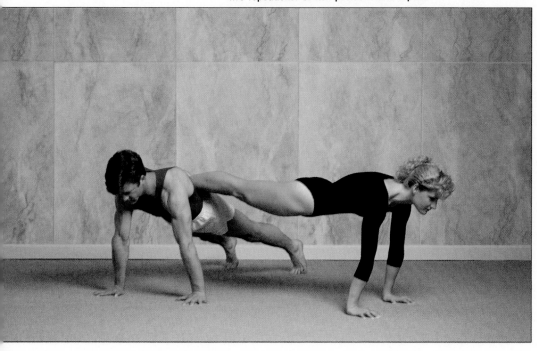

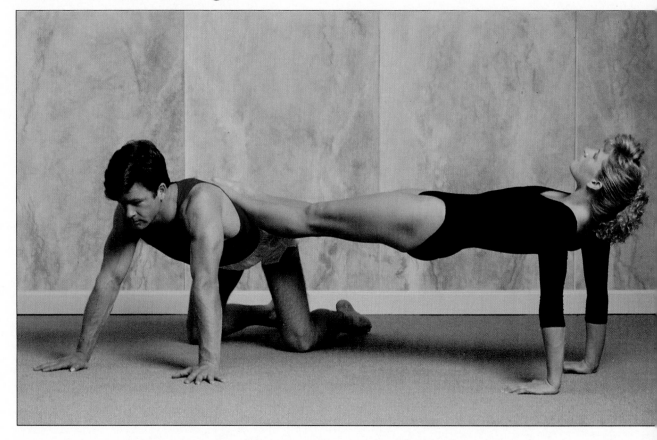

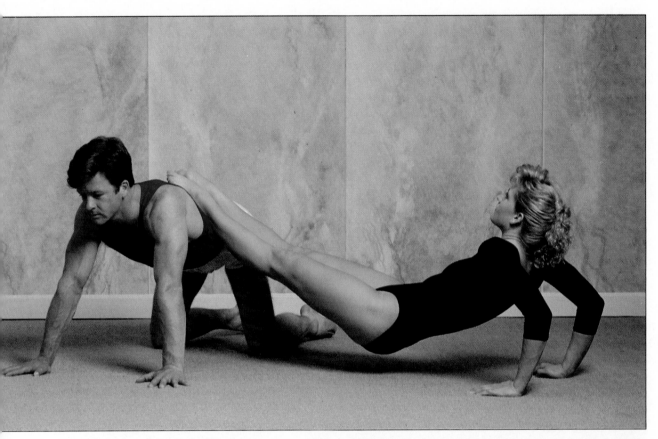

HE: Kneel on the floor on all fours. **SHE:** Keeping your legs and back straight, rest your calves on his back, and support yourself on your straight arms and hands *(above left).* **SHE:** Dip your hips until your buttocks are about four inches off the floor as you bend your elbows *(above).* Return to the starting position and repeat five times. For a variation: **SHE:** Dip your hips while keeping your arms straight *(right).* Return to the starting position.

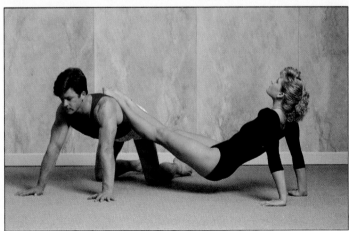

Balancing/1

The ability to keep your balance in unusual positions is one of the hardest skills to learn and maintain because it is used so rarely. The exercises on pages 106-123 are designed for practicing this skill in a progressively more advanced manner.

The first few exercises, the ones shown here and on pages 108-115, are the easiest. The later exercises, from page 116 to the end of the chapter, require more flexibility and strength to perform, as demonstrated in the photographs. Repeat all the movements, alternating right and left legs, where applicable, to develop balance evenly.

If your balancing and tumbling skills are not well developed, be particularly careful while doing the exercises on pages 120-123. Practice the basic balances, as well as the tumbling exercises in Chapter Three, and master them before attempting these last few movements. In particular, the exercise shown on pages 122-123 is the most difficult and challenging and should not be attempted by anyone who cannot comfortably perform all the other exercises in this book.

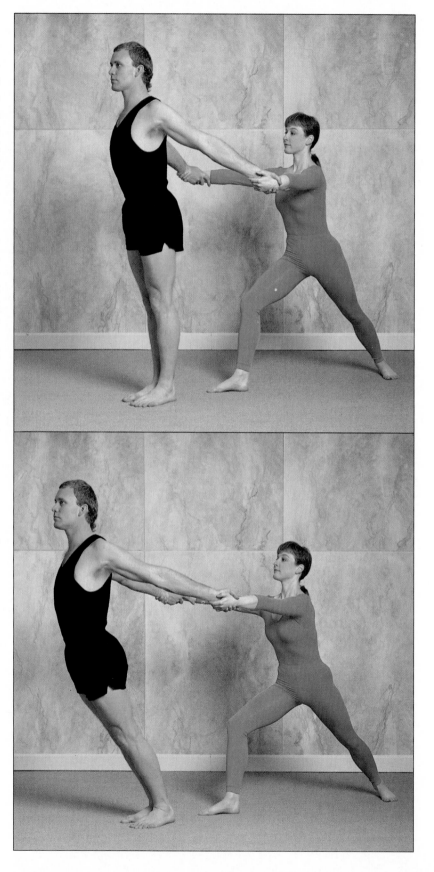

HE: Stand with your arms extended straight behind you. **SHE:** Stand behind your partner with one foot in front of the other, your front knee bent and hold his hands *(above right)*. **HE:** Lean forward, keeping your feet flat on the floor. **SHE:** Support your partner by holding onto his hands *(below right)*. Hold this position for 15 seconds. Return to the starting stance, switch positions and repeat.

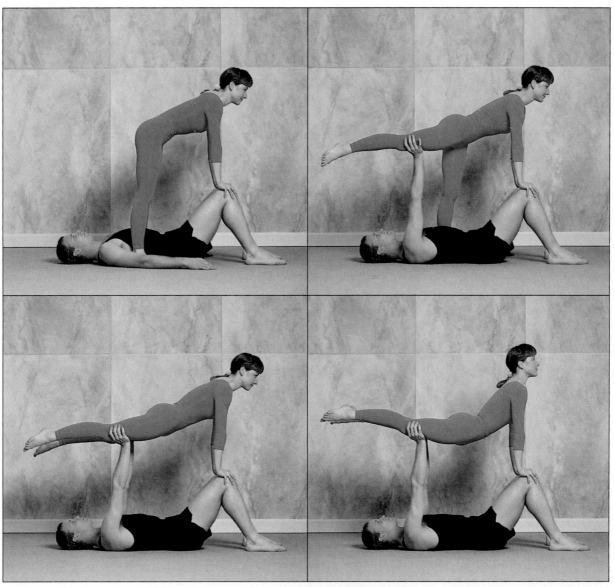

HE: Lie on your back with your arms straight at your sides, knees bent and feet flat on the floor. **SHE:** Stand with your feet on either side of his chest, lean forward and put your hands on his knees *(upper left)*. **SHE:** Extend your right leg straight backward. **HE:** Lift her right leg with your hand on her knee *(upper right)*. **SHE:** Extend your left leg back and keep your body straight. **HE:** Support the weight of her lower body with your hands on her knees, keeping your arms straight *(bottom left)*. **SHE:** Lift your head and arch your back slightly *(bottom right)*. Hold for 15 seconds, return to the starting position, switch positions and repeat.

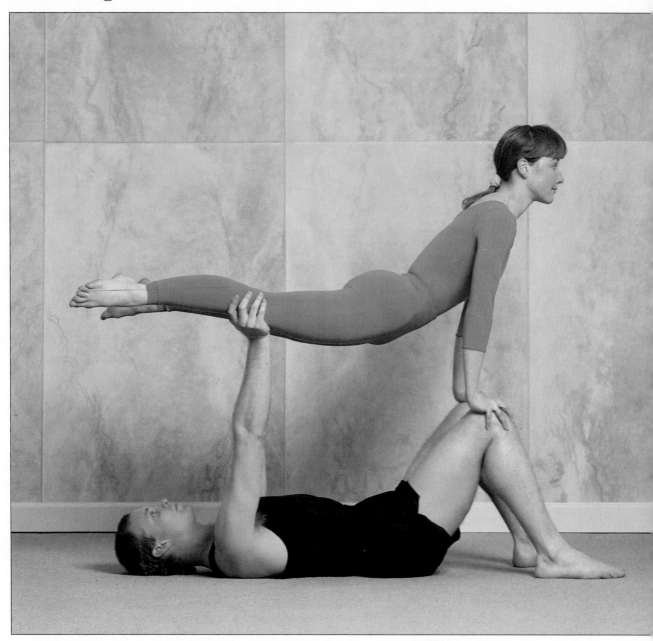

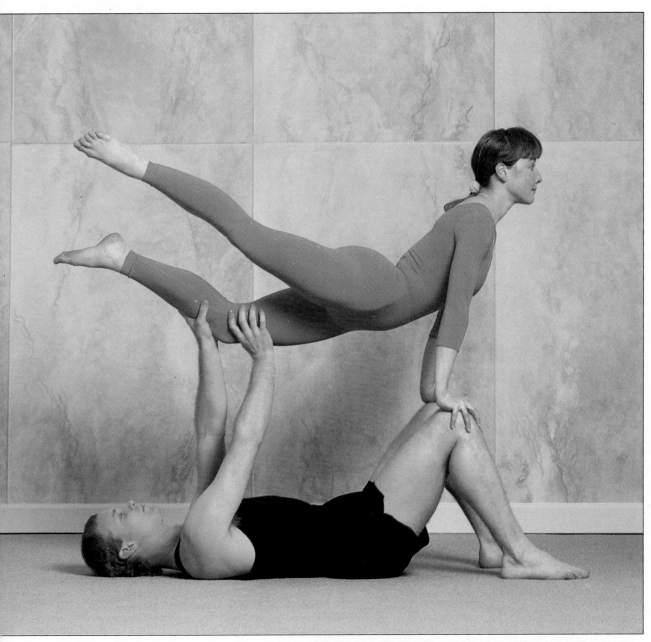

HE: Lie on your back with your knees bent and support her lower body by holding her knees with your hands. **SHE:** With your hands on his knees, arch your back as far as you can comfortably *(left)*. **SHE:** Lift your right leg, balance and hold for a moment *(right)*. Return to the starting position, switch positions and repeat.

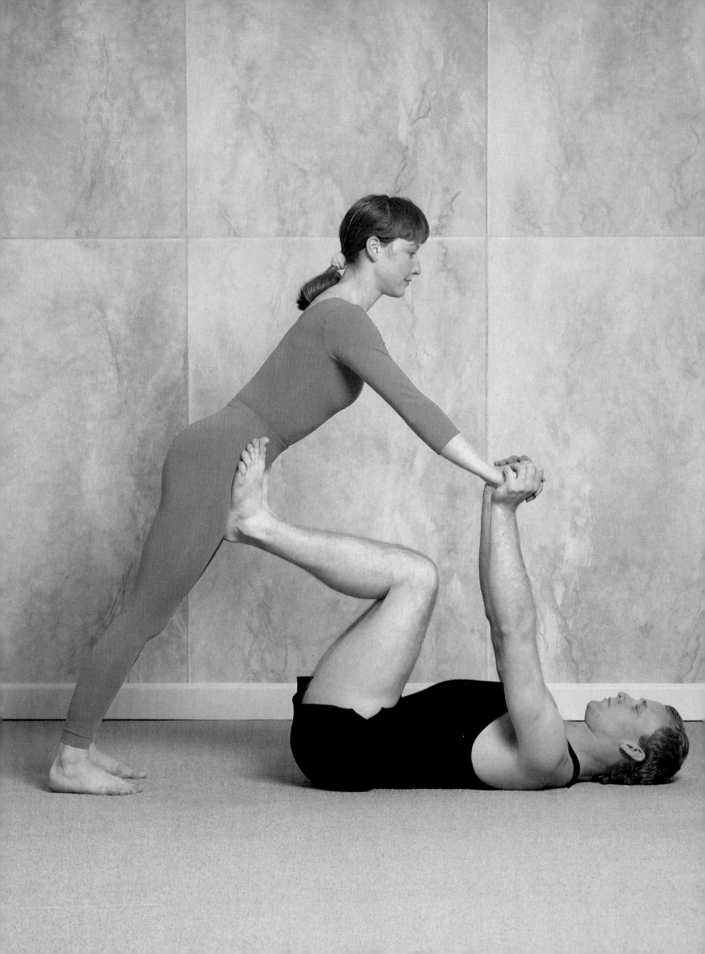

Balancing/3

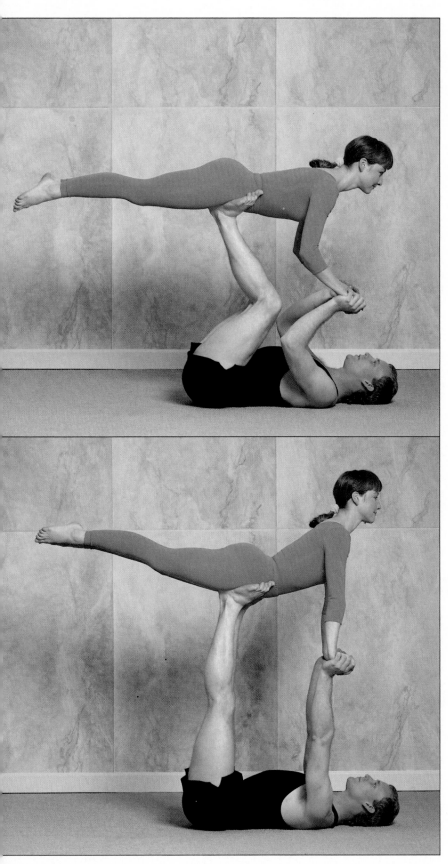

HE: Lie on your back with your knees bent and your feet off the ground. Hold her hands. **SHE:** Lean forward, bending slightly at the hips, hold his hands and rest your hips against his feet *(far left)*. **HE:** Pulling her arms toward you and supporting her with your feet, pull her forward until she is parallel to the floor. **SHE:** As you allow yourself to be lifted, keep your body straight *(left)*. **HE:** Straighten your legs and arms as you lift her up. **SHE:** Straighten your arms, raise your head and arch your back slightly *(below left)*. Hold for 15 seconds. Return to the starting position, then switch positions and repeat.

Balancing/4

SHE: Stand straight with your arms relaxed at your sides. **HE:** Stand behind your partner with your left hand around her waist *(below left)*. **SHE:** Lift your right leg outward to the side. **HE:** Support her right leg with your right arm, your hand under her knee *(below center)*. **SHE:** Lift your right leg outward as high and straight as possible. **HE:** Raise your left leg outward to the side as high and straight as possible *(right)*. **SHE:** Support his left leg with your left hand, and place your right hand under your right leg. Hold for 15 seconds, return to the starting position and repeat.

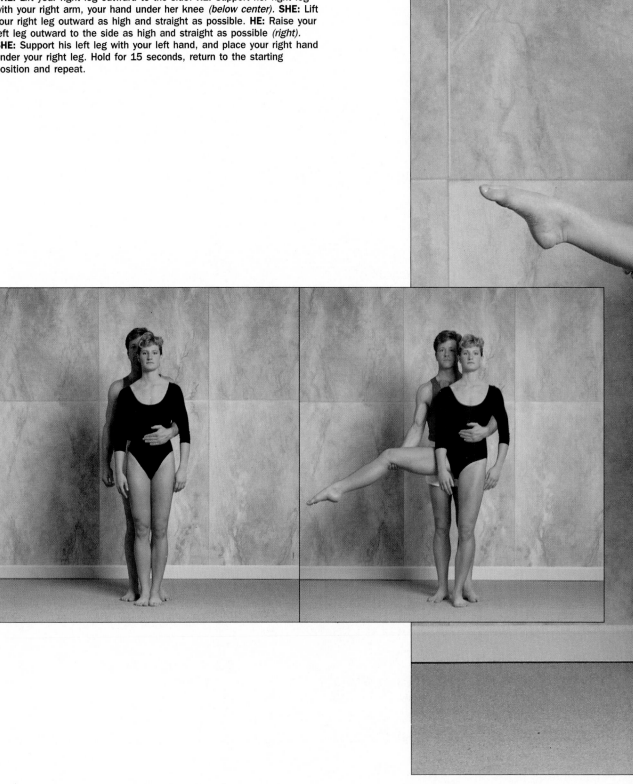

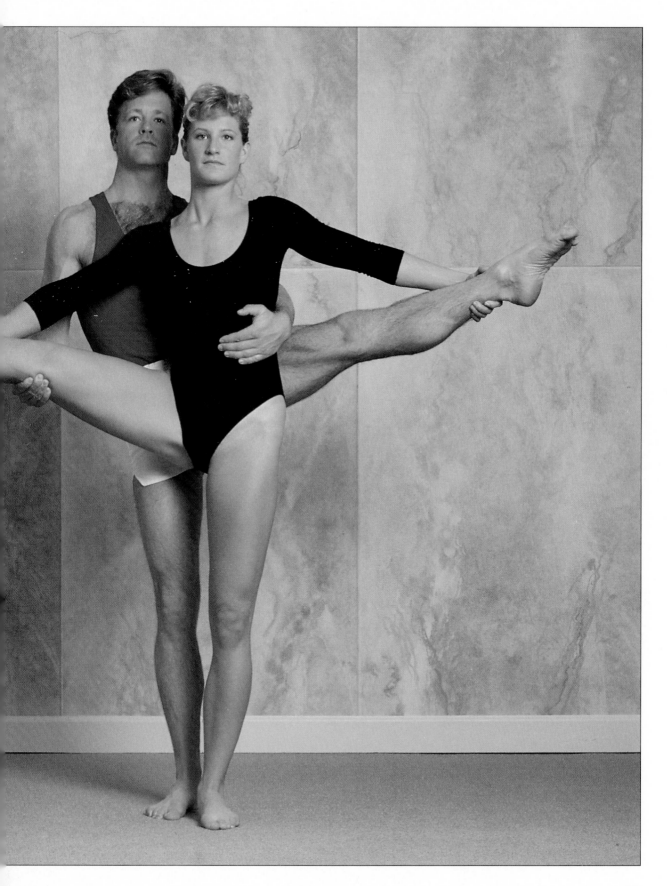

Balancing/5

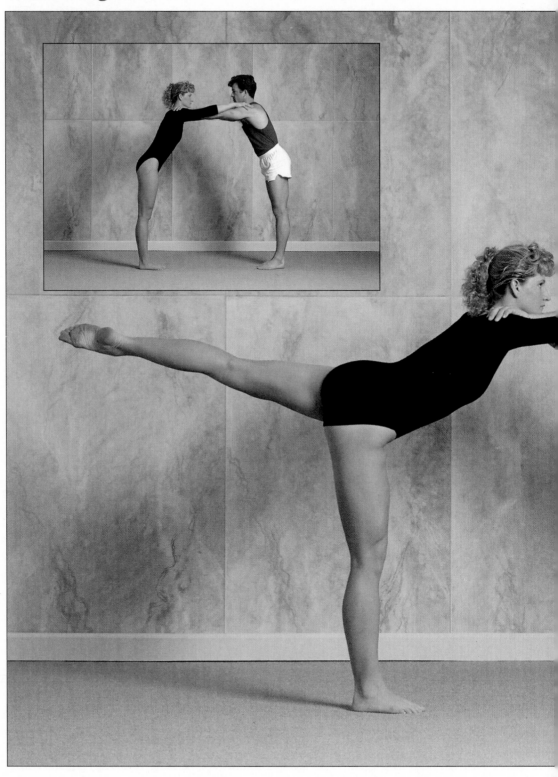

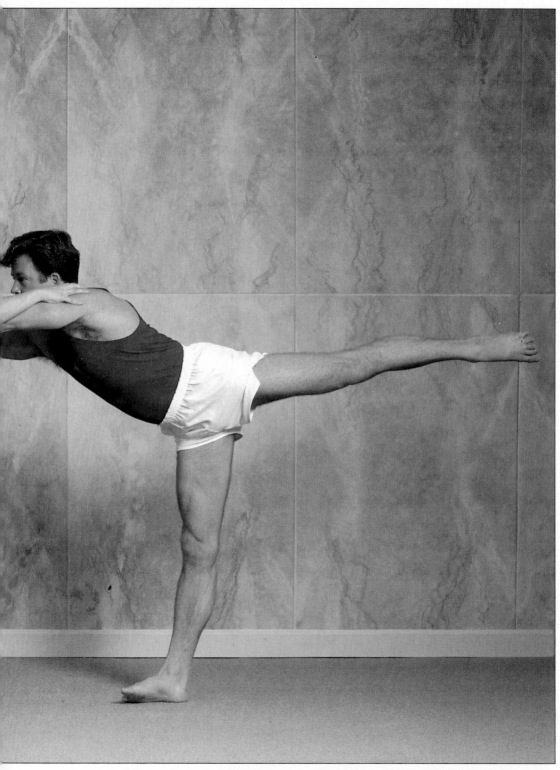

Both partners stand facing each other, bending forward slightly at the waist with hands on each others' shoulders *(inset)*. Both partners slowly raise their left feet backward as high and straight as possible *(above)*. Hold for 15 seconds, return to the starting position and repeat.

Balancing/6

HE: Kneel down on all fours. **SHE:** Lie with your back arched across his back, your arms extended over your head *(right).* **HE:** Lift your left leg backward and straighten your knee. **SHE:** Lift your right leg upward and straighten your knee *(above opposite).* **HE:** Extend your right arm forward *(below left).* Then return your right hand and left foot to the floor. **SHE:** Bring your knees toward your chest, reach your hands toward the outside of your ankles and lift your head *(below right).* Hold for 15 seconds, then switch positions and repeat.

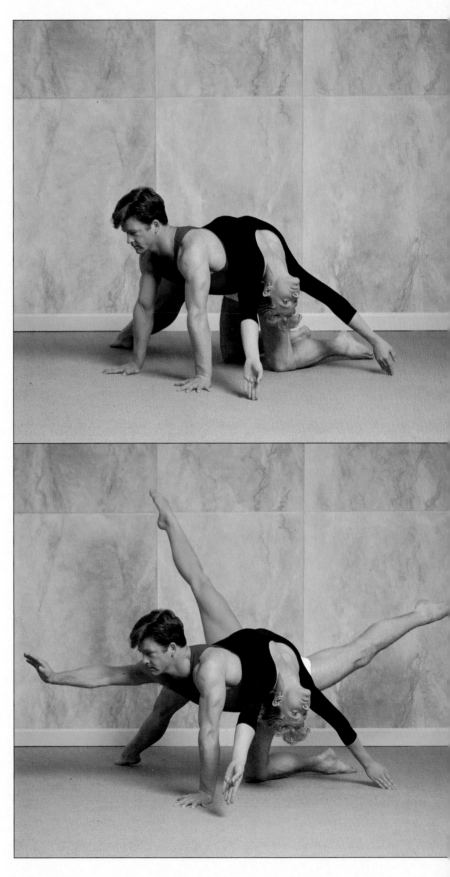

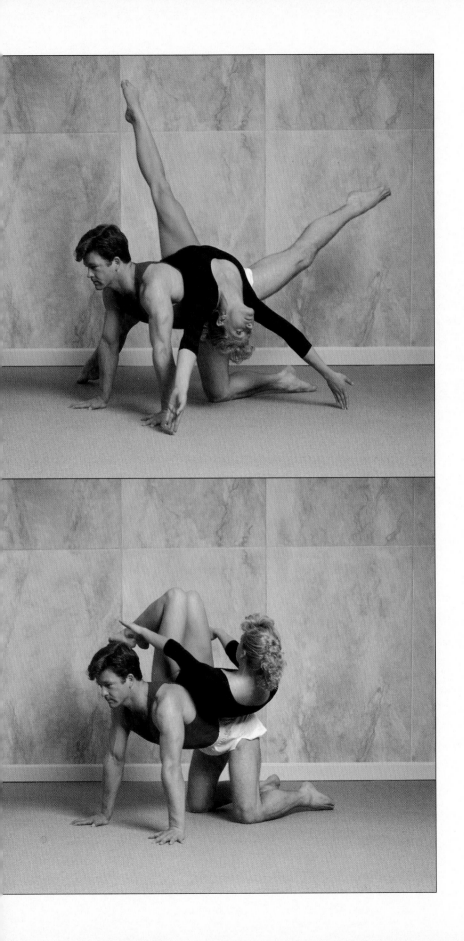

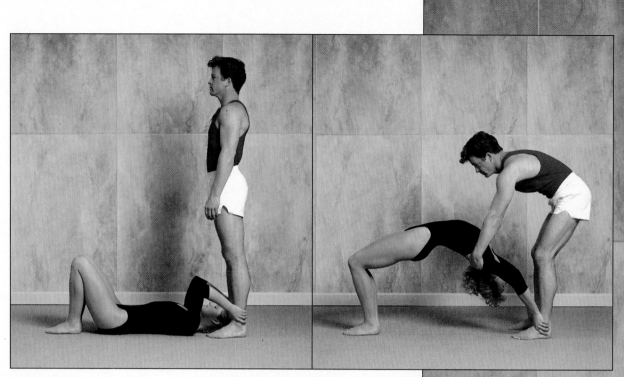

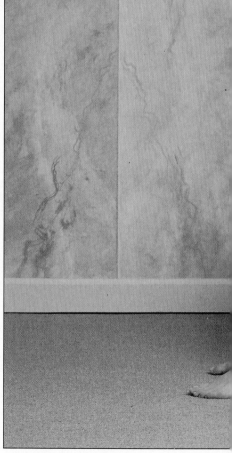

Balancing/7

SHE: Lie on your back with your knees bent, feet flat on the floor, elbows bent and hands grasping his ankles next to your head. **HE:** Stand with your feet on either side of her head *(above).* **SHE:** Arch your back off the floor. **HE:** Support her upper back and help her lift up *(above right).* **SHE:** Arch your back as high as possible. **HE:** Support her back without forcing her above her range of motion *(far right).* Switch positions and repeat.

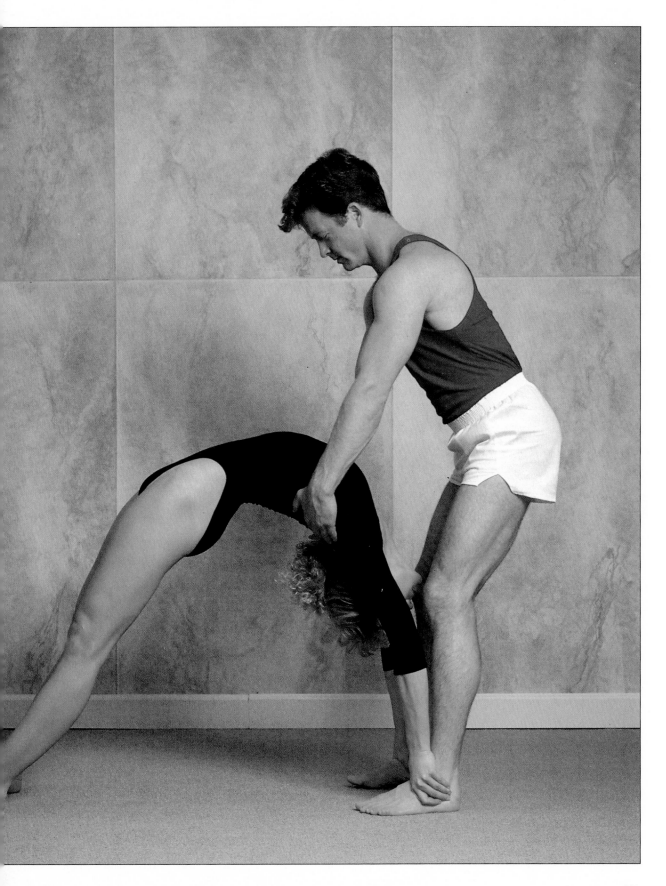

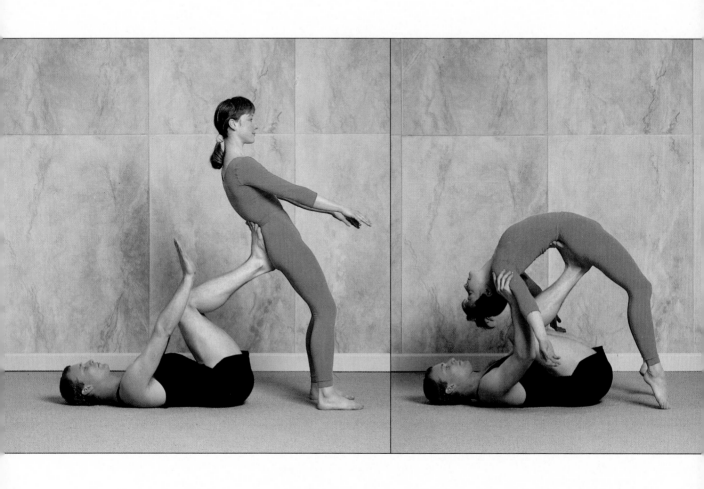

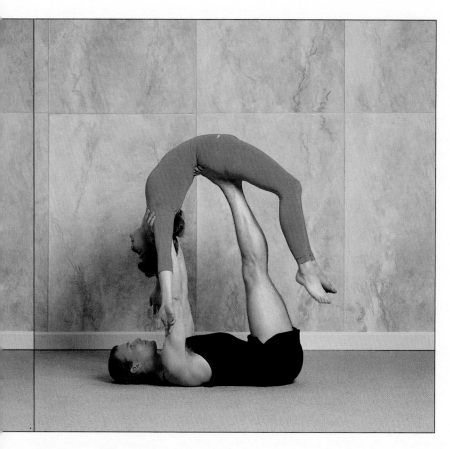

Balancing/8

HE: Lie on your back with your arms extended in front of your chest, knees bent, feet in the air at the level of your partner's lower back. **SHE:** Standing about a foot from your partner's buttocks, facing away from him, lean backward, allowing his feet to support your lower back and buttocks *(far left)*. **HE:** As your partner leans all the way backward, grasp her shoulders and bring your knees toward your chest until the top of her head is above your chin. **SHE:** Lean backward, keeping your body relaxed, your feet coming off the floor, your arms loose and outward to the sides *(center)*. **HE:** Support your partner in the air with your arms straight, your hands on her shoulders, your legs straight and your feet supporting her lower back. **SHE:** Let your body hang over your partner *(above)*. Hold for 15 seconds, switch positions and repeat.

Balancing/9

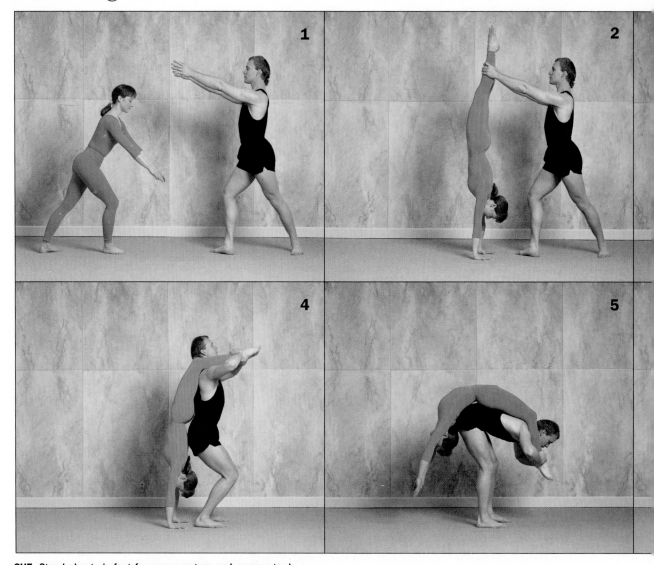

SHE: Stand about six feet from your partner and prepare to do a handstand. **HE:** Hold your arms in front of you to catch your partner's feet when she does a handstand (1). **SHE:** Perform a handstand. **HE:** Grasp her lower legs with both hands (2). **SHE:** Hold the handstand position. **HE:** Keeping a grip on her legs, turn and face away from her (3). **HE:** Bring your arms in front of you and pull her legs over your shoulders while you bend your knees (4). **HE:** Lean forward, keeping her weight on your back, and bring her feet toward the floor. **SHE:** Let your body hang loose and relaxed (5). **HE:** Place her feet flat on the floor. **SHE:** Keep your arms extended over your head and arch your back (6). **HE:** After releasing her ankles, begin to assume a standing position. **SHE:** Stand erect with your arms raised above your head *(far right)*.

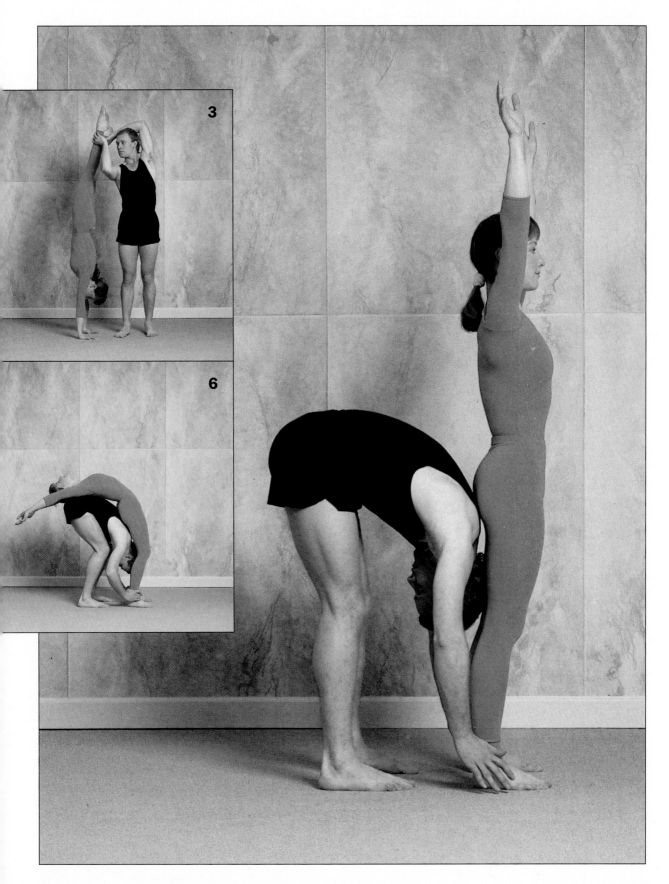

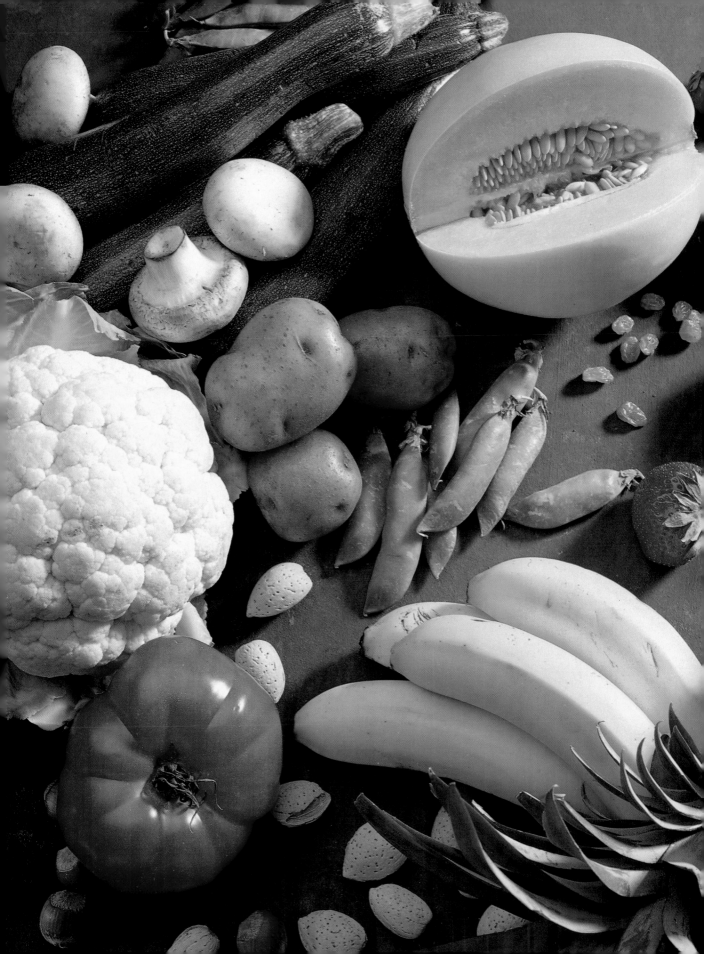

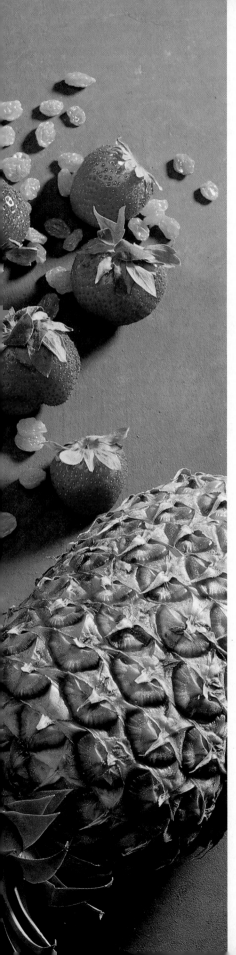

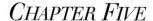

CHAPTER FIVE

Potassium and the Macrominerals

Regulating your muscles' release of energy

Potassium and the other major minerals — calcium, magnesium, chloride, phosphorus and sodium — are vital to coordinated muscle and nerve function. When you run, jump, tumble, throw or kick, the muscles and nerves must respond instantly to produce fast, powerful, accurate movement. Macro-minerals, as minerals required in the diet in relatively large amounts are called, make movement possible by transferring signals from the nerves to muscles, by working to release and store energy and by allowing muscle contraction to occur.

Potassium works in conjunction with sodium; the two minerals are balanced in all cells, and the signal from nerve to muscle travels across the cell membranes by means of a temporary change in this equilibrium. During contraction, potassium acts in the muscle tissue along with calcium to signal the small muscle units called myofibrils to move together. Then, along with magnesium, potassium acts as a muscle relaxant, causing the myofibrils to slide apart.

With phosphorus, potassium is required for releasing and storing energy. It is necessary for the breakdown of glucose — fuel — into energy, as well as for the transport of glucose across cell membranes. Potassium regulates the storage of glucose in the form of glycogen in muscle cells, especially in the rapid replacement of muscle glycogen after exercise. The stored glycogen cannot be converted directly back to glucose — the muscle lacks certain enzymes needed to make this possible — but the glycogen can be converted into lactic acid. Then, in the liver, potassium plays a significant role changing that lactic acid into glucose. In addition to performing these essential functions in muscle contraction and the release and storage of energy, potassium is necessary for nitrogen storage in protein synthesis.

Along with the other major minerals, potassium functions as an electrolyte, maintaining normal water balance, body temperature and blood pressure. The balance of electrical charges among the macro-minerals regulates how much fluid the body retains or loses. However, the regulation of body temperature through sweating, which is caused by the functioning of the electrolytes, may result in some electrolyte loss, especially during long workouts in warm temperatures. For this reason, it is important to eat foods that supply adequate macrominerals to avoid marginal deficiency, especially if you exercise.

The body works hard to maintain constant relative levels of macro-minerals and to avoid even small variations in their balance. As a result, significant potassium deficiency is very rare. When researchers have forced healthy subjects to sweat heavily over a period of days or weeks, they have not been able to induce potassium deficiency because the body will conserve this mineral when its reserves are low. However, in people who are already seriously ill or debilitated, po-tassium deficiency can cause hypokalemia, which results in muscle weakness and heart irregularities.

Recent studies indicate that inadequate intake of potassium may contribute to the development of hypertension. Doctors have always emphasized controlling sodium intake for lower blood pressure, but because of the precise balance between sodium and potassium, researchers have become interested in the possible protective effect of increased potassium intake. Data analyzed from the first National Health and Nutrition Examination Survey (HANES) showed a corre-lation between inadequate potassium levels and increased systolic blood pressure.

Adequate potassium intake may protect against stroke and high systolic blood pressure. A recent study of 859 men and women over a 12-year period, reported in the *New England Journal of Medicine,* found that subjects with a higher dietary potassium intake had a lower incidence of mortality from stroke. Subjects who increased their con-sumption of potassium-rich food by approximately one serving of fruit or vegetables daily showed a 40 percent reduction in stroke.

Because potassium is found in so many fresh foods, deficiency in a

The Basic Guidelines

For a moderately active adult, the National Institutes of Health recommends a diet that is low in fat, high in carbohydrates and moderate in protein. The institutes' guidelines suggest that no more than 30 percent of your calories come from fat, that 55 to 60 percent come from carbohydrates and that no more than 15 percent come from protein. A gram of fat equals nine calories, while a gram of protein or carbohydrate equals four calories; therefore, if you eat 2,100 calories a day, you should consume approximately 60 grams of fat, 315 grams of carbohydrate and no more than 75 grams of protein daily. If you follow a lowfat/high-carbohydrate diet, your chance of developing heart disease, cancer and other life-threatening diseases may be considerably reduced.

◆ The nutrition charts that accompany each of the lowfat/high-carbohydrate recipes in this book include the number of calories per serving, the number of grams of fat, carbohydrate and protein in a serving, and the percentage of calories derived from each of these nutrients. In addition, the charts provide the amount of calcium, iron and sodium per serving.

◆ Calcium deficiency may be associated with periodontal disease — which attacks the mouth's bones and tissues, including the gums — in both men and women, and with osteoporosis, or bone shrinking and weakening, in the elderly. The deficiency may also contribute to high blood pressure. The recommended daily allowance for calcium is 800 milligrams a day for men and women. Pregnant and lactating women are advised to consume 1,200 milligrams daily; a National Institutes of Health consensus panel recommends that postmenopausal women consume 1,200 to 1,500 milligrams of calcium daily.

◆ Although one way you can reduce your fat intake is to cut your consumption of red meat, you should make sure that you get your necessary iron from other sources. The Food and Nutrition Board of the National Academy of Sciences suggests a minimum of 10 milligrams of iron per day for men and 18 milligrams for women between the ages of 11 and 50.

◆ High sodium intake is associated with high blood pressure. Most adults should restrict sodium intake to between 2,000 and 2,500 milligrams a day, according to the National Academy of Sciences. One way to keep sodium consumption in check is not to add table salt to food.

well-balanced diet is unlikely. No recommended daily allowance has yet been established, but the Food and Nutrition Board has estimated a safe and adequate range of 1,500-6,000 milligrams per day. The safest source is food. Unless your doctor advises it, do not take potassium supplements: Excess potassium can cause the heart to dilate and become flaccid, slowing its rate. In addition to vegetables, fruits and whole-grain cereals are some of the best sources of potassium, and milk, meat, fish, legumes and nuts are also good. Avoid highly processed convenience and snack foods, which lose their potassium during preparation; they are also excessively high in sodium.

The dishes in this chapter combine foods that are naturally rich in potassium and low in sodium. The Sweet Potato-Banana Pudding on page 139 contains 640 milligrams of potassium and only 13 milligrams of sodium and the Oranges with Three-Fruit Sauce contains 835 milligrams of potassium and 46 milligrams of sodium per serving.

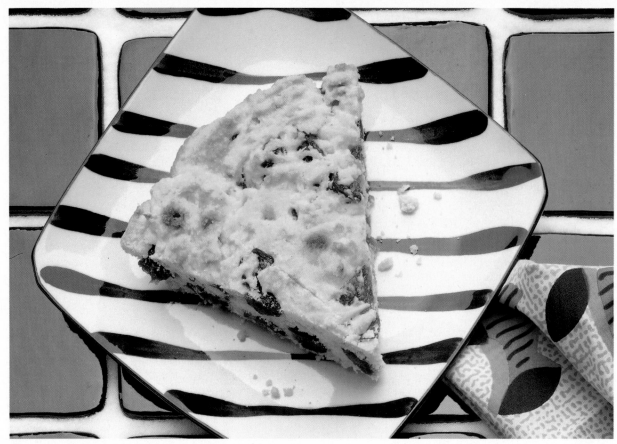

Skillet Cornbread with Prunes

Breakfast
· · · · · · · · · · · · · · · · · · · ·

SKILLET CORNBREAD WITH PRUNES

Prunes are rich sources of potassium and iron. Baking them in bread preserves more of their mineral content than cooking them in liquid.

CALORIES per serving	267
68% Carbohydrate	46 g
8% Protein	6 g
24% Fat	7 g
CALCIUM	128 mg
IRON	2 mg
SODIUM	245 mg

1/4 cup margarine
1 1/2 cups unbleached
  all-purpose flour
1/2 cup yellow cornmeal
1/4 cup brown sugar

2 1/2 teaspoons baking powder
1 egg, lightly beaten
1 cup buttermilk
1 cup coarsely chopped
  pitted prunes

Preheat the oven to 375° F. Melt the margarine in a 9-inch ovenproof nonstick skillet over medium-low heat. Meanwhile, in a medium-size bowl combine the flour, cornmeal, sugar and baking powder, and make a well in the center. Swirl the skillet to coat it completely with margarine, then pour the margarine into the well in the dry ingredients (leave a coating of margarine on the skillet). Add the egg, buttermilk and prunes, and stir just until the dry ingredients are incorporated. Turn the batter into the skillet, spread it evenly with a spatula and bake for 30 minutes, or until the bread is golden on top and a toothpick inserted into the center comes out clean and dry.   Makes 8 servings

BULGUR-BANANA PORRIDGE

Bulgur, a popular cereal in the Middle East, consists of kernels of whole wheat that have been steamed and then crushed. Bulgur supplies more potassium than oatmeal and makes a pleasant change for breakfast. The milk in the porridge, and the almonds that top it, contribute calcium, which works with potassium to make muscles contract.

CALORIES per serving	235
70% Carbohydrate	42 g
15% Protein	9 g
15% Fat	4 g
CALCIUM	185 mg
IRON	2 mg
SODIUM	83 mg

2 bananas

1 egg, lightly beaten

1 tablespoon pure maple syrup

2 teaspoons cornstarch

1/2 teaspoon vanilla extract

1/4 teaspoon ground nutmeg

1/4 teaspoon ground cinnamon

1/2 cup bulgur

2 cups skim milk

1/2 ounce toasted almonds, slivered

Preheat the oven to 325°F. Peel and mash the bananas and place them in a medium-size saucepan. Add the egg, maple syrup, cornstarch, vanilla, nutmeg and cinnamon, and stir well. Add the bulgur, then gradually stir in the milk. Bring the mixture to a boil over medium-high heat and cook, stirring constantly, for 1 minute, or until well blended and thickened. Transfer the porridge to a 1-quart baking dish and bake it for 25 minutes, or until set. Stir the porridge, divide it among 4 bowls and top each portion with almonds.

Makes 4 servings

ORANGES WITH THREE-FRUIT SAUCE

This dish is a more than adequate substitute for drinking a glass of juice at breakfast. A serving of the combination of fruits, milk and nuts supplies almost twice as much potassium as an 8-ounce glass of orange or grapefruit juice— and slightly more vitamin C.

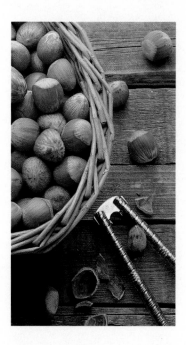

1/2 cup unsweetened apple juice

1/3 cup dried apricots

4 large navel oranges

1 1/2 cups cantaloupe chunks

1/2 cup fresh or frozen raspberries

1/2 cup evaporated skimmed milk

1 ounce toasted hazelnuts, chopped

Place the apple juice and apricots in a small saucepan and bring to a boil over medium-high heat. Reduce the heat to low and simmer, partially covered, for 10 minutes, or until the apricots are soft. Meanwhile, peel and section the oranges, removing the membranes; set aside.

For the sauce, transfer the apricots and their cooking liquid to a food processor or blender and process for 5 to 10 seconds, or until puréed, scraping down the sides of the container with a rubber spatula. Add the cantaloupe and process until puréed, then add the raspberries and process until puréed. Add 1/4 cup of milk and process for 5 seconds, or until the sauce is blended and slightly thickened, then stir in the remaining milk. Divide the sauce among 4 bowls and top it with the orange sections. Sprinkle each portion with hazelnuts and serve.

Makes 4 servings

CALORIES per serving	217
71% Carbohydrate	42 g
10% Protein	6 g
19% Fat	5 g
CALCIUM	191 mg
IRON	1 mg
SODIUM	46 mg

GINGER SCONES

CALORIES per scone	241
65% Carbohydrate	39 g
9% Protein	6 g
26% Fat	7 g
CALCIUM	121 mg
IRON	2 mg
SODIUM	270 mg

Adding whole-wheat flour to baked goods greatly enhances their nutritional value. When grain products are refined, the outer layer of the seed is removed. Whole-wheat flour retains its bran, which is a rich source of potassium, magnesium and phosphorus.

1 1/2 cups unbleached
  all-purpose flour
1/2 cup whole-wheat flour
2 tablespoons sugar
2 teaspoons baking powder
Pinch of salt
3 tablespoons plus
  1 teaspoon margarine

1 tablespoon plus 1 teaspoon
  crystallized ginger, finely
  chopped (1/2 ounce)
2 teaspoons grated orange peel
1/4 teaspoon ground ginger
2/3 cup buttermilk

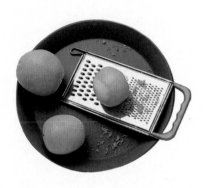

Preheat the oven to 425° F. Combine the all-purpose flour, whole-wheat flour, sugar, baking powder and salt in a food processor. Add the margarine and process, pulsing the machine on and off, for 5 to 10 seconds, or until the mixture resembles coarse cornmeal. Add the crystallized ginger, orange peel and ground ginger, then with the machine running, add the buttermilk and process until the dough begins to clump together. Knead the dough briefly by hand until it is smooth. (To mix the dough by hand, stir together the dry ingredients in a large bowl. Using a pastry blender or 2 knives, cut in the margarine until the mixture resembles coarse cornmeal. Stir in the remaining ingredients, then knead until smooth.) Divide the dough into 6 equal pieces (do not roll them into smooth balls), place them on a baking sheet and lightly shape them into mounds. Bake the scones for 12 to 15 minutes, or until they are golden brown on top. Serve warm.   Makes 6 scones

STRAWBERRY-APPLE SHAKE

CALORIES per serving	255
76% Carbohydrate	50 g
19% Protein	12 g
5% Fat	2 g
CALCIUM	263 mg
IRON	1 mg
SODIUM	277 mg

Dairy products and fruits eaten at breakfast can supply much of the calcium and potassium you need daily. This creamy fruit shake gives you about one third of the calcium you need daily; it also provides about half the estimated requirement of potassium and all the vitamin C requirement.

1 cup fresh or unsweetened
  strawberries
3 tablespoons lowfat
  cottage cheese (1%)

1/4 cup unsweetened frozen
  apple juice concentrate
1 teaspoon vanilla extract
2/3 cup skim milk

If using fresh strawberries, wash, hull and halve them. Place the strawberries in a plastic bag and freeze them for 3 hours, or until they are frozen solid. If using frozen strawberries, thaw them just enough to break them apart for measuring, then return them to the freezer until frozen solid.

Place the cottage cheese in a blender and process it for 5 to 10 seconds, or until smooth. Add the apple juice and process for 5 seconds more. Add the strawberries and vanilla and process for 15 seconds, or until the strawberries are puréed. Add the milk and process for another 5 seconds, or until well blended. Pour the shake into a tall glass and serve.   Makes 1 serving

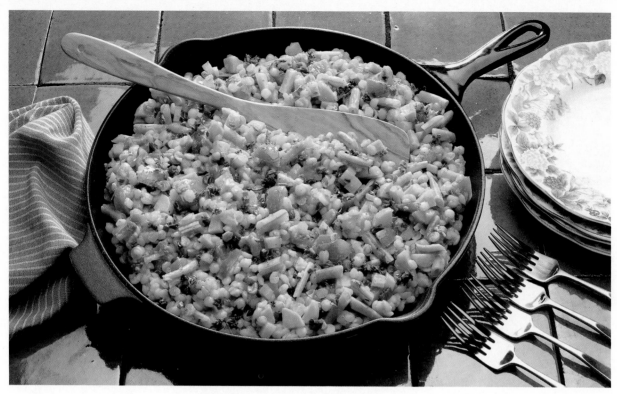

Lentil Pilaf

Lunch
············

LENTIL PILAF

A strong, lean body is essential for a gymnast, and an asset to any athlete. Cutting calories can mean losing nutrients as well, but this lowfat meal is an excellent source of iron, potassium and vitamin A.

CALORIES per serving	272
54% Carbohydrate	38 g
22% Protein	16 g
24% Fat	8 g
CALCIUM	75 mg
IRON	6 mg
SODIUM	162 mg

1 cup yellow lentils
2 teaspoons turmeric
2 tablespoons safflower oil
2 garlic cloves, finely chopped
1/2 pound fresh tomatoes, coarsely chopped
1 cup coarsely chopped carrots
1 cup coarsely chopped green beans
1 cup coarsely chopped scallions
2 tablespoons chopped fresh parsley
3/4 teaspoon ground cumin
1/4 teaspoon salt

Place the lentils and 1 teaspoon of turmeric in a medium-size saucepan with 2 cups of water and bring to a boil over medium-high heat. Cover the pan, reduce the heat to low and simmer for 30 minutes, or until the lentils are just tender; set aside to keep warm.

Heat 1 tablespoon of oil in a medium-size nonstick skillet over medium-high heat. Add the garlic and sauté for 30 seconds, or just until fragrant. Add the tomatoes, carrots, green beans, scallions, parsley, cumin and salt, and cook, stirring frequently, for 5 minutes, or until the vegetables just begin to color. Add the lentils and any liquid in the saucepan, the remaining oil and turmeric, and cook, stirring, for another 5 minutes, or until the lentils are heated through and the vegetables are crisp-tender.   Makes 4 servings

TOFU HUMMUS WITH PITA CRISPS

Dips made from cheese or sour cream are rich in calcium but can be very high in saturated fat. This version of hummus is made with tofu, sesame seeds and broccoli, which are among the best nondairy sources of dietary calcium.

CALORIES per serving	236
60% Carbohydrate	36 g
20% Protein	12 g
20% Fat	5 g
CALCIUM	141 mg
IRON	3 mg
SODIUM	293 mg

3 squares firm tofu (3/4 pound), quartered
1 cup cooked, drained chickpeas
3 tablespoons lemon juice
1 tablespoon tahini (sesame paste)
1 garlic clove, peeled and crushed
2 tablespoons chopped fresh dill
Six 1-ounce pita breads
1 medium-size sweet potato, boiled, cooled and peeled
1/4 teaspoon salt
Ground pepper
1 1/2 teaspoons sesame seeds
1 1/2 cups broccoli florets, blanched and cooled

Place the tofu in a food processor or blender with the chickpeas, lemon juice, tahini and garlic, and process until smooth. Transfer the mixture to a serving bowl, stir in the dill, cover and refrigerate.

Preheat the oven to 350° F. Split the pita breads and cut each piece into quarters. Spread the pieces on a baking sheet and toast them for 10 minutes, or until lightly browned around the edges. Meanwhile, cut the sweet potato into finger-length sticks. To serve, season the hummus with salt, and pepper to taste. Divide it among 6 plates and sprinkle each portion with sesame seeds. Arrange the broccoli florets, sweet potato sticks and pita triangles around the hummus and serve.　　Makes 6 servings

COLD PEANUT PASTA

Although the fat in peanut butter is mostly mono- and polyunsaturated, it is still a high-fat product and should not be a mainstay of your diet. However, peanut butter is an excellent source of potassium and, when combined with a grain product like pasta, provides a complete protein.

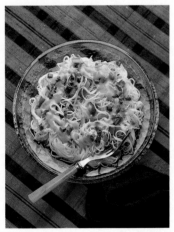

CALORIES per serving	366
57% Carbohydrate	53 g
13% Protein	12 g
30% Fat	13 g
CALCIUM	39 mg
IRON	3 mg
SODIUM	592 mg

1/2 pound capellini or spaghettini
3 tablespoons smooth peanut butter
1 tablespoon plus 2 teaspoons Oriental sesame oil
2 tablespoons soy sauce
1 tablespoon rice vinegar
2 teaspoons brown sugar
1/4 teaspoon hot pepper sauce
1 cup shredded carrots
1 cup diced green bell pepper
1/2 cup chopped scallions
2 tablespoons chopped fresh coriander or parsley

Bring a large pot of water to a boil. Cook the pasta for 8 minutes, or according to the package directions, until al dente. Drain the pasta in a colander, rinse it under cold running water and set aside in the colander to drain again. Meanwhile, for the sauce, in a small bowl stir together the peanut butter and oil until blended. Gradually add the soy sauce, vinegar, sugar, hot pepper sauce and 2 tablespoons of water, and stir until smoothly blended.

Transfer the pasta to a serving bowl, add the carrots, bell pepper and scallions and toss well. Pour on the sauce and sprinkle with the coriander. If not serving immediately, cover and refrigerate the pasta.　　Makes 4 servings

BLACK-EYED PEA SOUP

This soup offers about three times the potassium and one third the sodium of canned pea soup with ham.

1 cup dried black-eyed peas	1 cup diced celery
2 tablespoons plus	1 cup frozen lima beans
2 teaspoons margarine	1/2 cup low-sodium chicken stock
1 cup chopped onion	1 teaspoon ground cumin
2 garlic cloves, chopped	1 teaspoon coriander seeds
One 14-ounce can plum tomatoes	1/4 teaspoon black pepper
1 cup diced carrots	

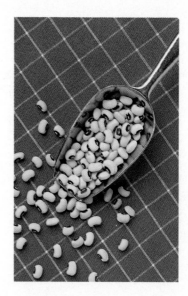

Place the peas in a medium-size bowl with cold water to cover by 2 inches. Let the peas soak overnight in the refrigerator.

Drain the peas and set aside. Melt the margarine in a large saucepan over medium-high heat. Add the onion and garlic, and sauté for 2 to 3 minutes, or until the onions begin to turn translucent. Add the peas, the tomatoes with their juice, the carrots, celery, lima beans, stock, cumin, coriander, pepper and 1 cup of water, and stir to combine. Bring the mixture to a boil, then cover the pan, reduce the heat to low and simmer for 30 minutes.

Using a slotted spoon, transfer about two thirds of the solids from the soup to a food processor or blender, and purée. Return the purée to the saucepan and stir to blend it. Bring the soup to a boil over medium-high heat and simmer it, stirring constantly, for 2 minutes, or until heated through. Ladle the soup into 4 bowls and serve.   Makes 4 servings

CALORIES per serving	314
57% Carbohydrate	46 g
18% Protein	15 g
25% Fat	9 g
CALCIUM	125 mg
IRON	6 mg
SODIUM	328 mg

TURKEY TETRAZZINI

Using onions, fresh herbs and small amounts of flavorful cheese as seasonings helps you eliminate the salt from many recipes.

1 cup low-sodium chicken stock	1 tablespoon plus
1 1/2 cups sliced	2 teaspoons cornstarch
fresh mushrooms	2 ounces skinless cooked turkey
1 cup chopped red onion	1 cup frozen peas
1 cup frozen corn kernels	1/4 cup chopped fresh parsley
1/3 cup skim milk	1/2 pound fettuccine
1 tablespoon sherry	2 tablespoons grated Parmesan

Bring the stock to a boil in a medium-size saucepan over medium-high heat. Add the mushrooms, onion and corn, reduce the heat to medium and simmer the mixture for 8 to 10 minutes, or until the mushrooms are tender. Meanwhile, in a small bowl stir together the milk, sherry and cornstarch until well blended. Cut the turkey into cubes. Bring the stock to a boil, stir in the cornstarch mixture and boil for 2 minutes, or until the sauce thickens. Add the turkey, peas and parsley, remove the pan from the heat, cover and set aside to keep warm.

Bring a large pot of water to a boil, add the fettuccine and cook for 10 minutes, or according to the package directions, until al dente; drain and transfer to a serving bowl. Stir in the turkey mixture and toss until combined, then sprinkle the mixture with Parmesan and serve.   Makes 6 servings

CALORIES per serving	239
73% Carbohydrate	44 g
19% Protein	12 g
8% Fat	2 g
CALCIUM	69 mg
IRON	2 mg
SODIUM	85 mg

Dinner

CAULIFLOWER-PARSLEY SALAD WITH CHICKEN

Parsley is more than just a garnish — it is an excellent source of potassium and vitamins A and C. Cauliflower belongs to the family of cruciferous plants, which also includes broccoli and cabbage. These vegetables are high in fiber and vitamin C.

CALORIES per serving	361
54% Carbohydrate	49 g
16% Protein	15 g
30% Fat	12 g
CALCIUM	99 mg
IRON	4 mg
SODIUM	517 mg

1/4 pound boneless,
  skinless chicken breast
2 1/4 cups cauliflower florets
1/2 cup rice vinegar
3 tablespoons walnut oil
2 teaspoons Worcestershire
  sauce
1 teaspoon sugar

1 tablespoon chopped
  fresh tarragon, or 1 teaspoon
  dried tarragon
1/4 teaspoon salt
1/4 teaspoon pepper
1 papaya (about 3/4 pound)
1/2 pound tomatoes
2 cups packed parsley, trimmed
6 ounces breadsticks

Bring 2 cups of water to a boil over medium-high heat in a small saucepan. Add the chicken, reduce the heat to low, partially cover the pan and simmer for 10 minutes, or until the chicken is firm and the juices run clear when pierced with

Cauliflower-Parsley Salad with Chicken

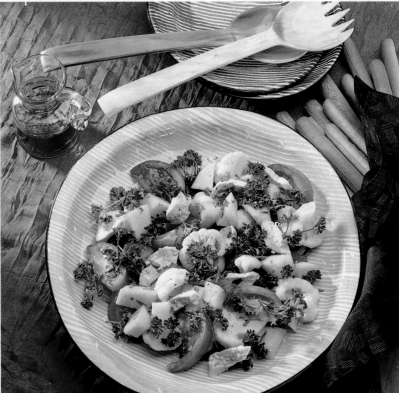

134

the tip of a knife. Transfer the chicken to a plate, cover loosely with plastic wrap and set aside to cool.

Bring a medium-size saucepan of water to a boil. Blanch the cauliflower in the boiling water for 2 to 4 minutes, or until it is tender when pierced with a knife. Drain the cauliflower, cool under cold running water and set aside to drain again.

For the dressing, in a small bowl stir together the vinegar, oil, Worcestershire sauce, sugar, tarragon, salt and pepper; set aside. Peel and seed the papaya and cut it into 1-inch cubes. Halve and core the tomatoes, then cut them into 1/2-inch-thick wedges. When the chicken is cool, cut it on the diagonal into 1/4-inch-thick slices. Place the cauliflower, parsley, papaya, tomatoes and chicken in a large bowl. Stir the dressing to recombine it. Pour the dressing over the salad, toss it gently and serve it with the breadsticks.

Makes 4 servings

CARIBBEAN SEAFOOD CHOWDER

Minerals are lost when produce is cooked in water, especially if the liquid is discarded after cooking; potassium is particularly susceptible. The fruits and vegetables in this recipe are cooked for only ten minutes in their own juices, which form the "stock" for the chowder.

CALORIES per serving	487
63% Carbohydrate	79 g
14% Protein	17 g
23% Fat	13 g
CALCIUM	115 mg
IRON	4 mg
SODIUM	372 mg

1 cup brown rice
3 tablespoons plus
   2 teaspoons margarine
2 cups chopped leeks
2 garlic cloves, chopped
2 tablespoons unbleached
   all-purpose flour
One 14-ounce can peeled
   plum tomatoes
1/4 pound scallops
1/4 pound filet of sole, cut into
   1-inch pieces

1 cup green beans, cut in
   1-inch pieces
1 cup juice-packed pineapple
   chunks, drained, 1/2 cup of
   juice reserved
1/2 jalapeño pepper, seeded
2 teaspoons brown sugar
2 bananas, peeled and
   cut into chunks
Pinch of Cayenne pepper

Bring 2 cups of water to a boil in a medium-size saucepan over medium-high heat. Stir in the rice. Cover the pan, reduce the heat to medium-low and simmer for 40 minutes, or until the rice is tender and the water is absorbed.

Ten minutes before the rice is done, melt 1 teaspoon of margarine in a large nonstick skillet over medium-high heat. Add the leeks and garlic, and sauté for 2 minutes, or until the leeks are limp. Transfer the leeks and garlic to a bowl and set aside. Melt the remaining margarine over medium heat and stir in the flour until blended, then slowly stir in the tomatoes and their liquid. Bring the mixture to a boil and cook for 1 to 2 minutes, or until slightly thickened. Add the scallops, sole, green beans, pineapple chunks and juice, jalapeño and sugar, and return the mixture to a boil. Cover the pan, reduce the heat to low and simmer for 5 minutes, or until the fish turns opaque and the vegetables are tender. Add the leeks and garlic, the bananas and Cayenne, and cook, stirring, for 1 minute more, or until the fish flakes when tested with a knife and all of the ingredients are heated through. Remove and discard the jalapeño. Divide the rice among 4 bowls, top it with the chowder and serve.

Makes 4 servings

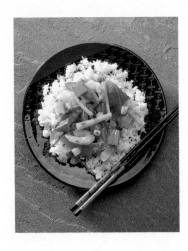

SZECHUAN SHRIMP AND VEGETABLES

This Chinese-style dinner is an especially rich source of minerals and vitamins: Shrimp and rice supply magnesium and iron, while the vegetables provide potassium and all the vitamins A and C you need each day.

1 cup white rice	2 tablespoons slivered ginger
1/4 cup low-sodium chicken stock	3 garlic cloves, chopped
1 tablespoon sherry	6 ounces shelled shrimp
1 tablespoon soy sauce	1 cup julienned carrots
2 teaspoons brown sugar	1 1/2 cups diced red bell pepper
2 teaspoons cornstarch	1/4 pound snow peas, trimmed
3 tablespoons plus 1 teaspoon	1 cup chopped scallions
vegetable oil	1/4 teaspoon red pepper flakes

Bring 2 cups of water to a boil in a medium-size saucepan over medium-high heat. Stir in the rice. Cover the pan, reduce the heat to medium-low and simmer for 20 minutes, or until the rice is tender and the water is absorbed. Meanwhile, in a small bowl stir together the stock, sherry, soy sauce, sugar, cornstarch and 1/4 cup of water, and set aside.

Heat 1 tablespoon of oil in a large nonstick skillet over medium-high heat. Add half of the ginger and garlic, and stir fry for 5 seconds. Add the shrimp and stir fry for 2 to 3 minutes, or until the shrimp turn almost completely orange. Transfer the mixture to a bowl, cover loosely with foil and set aside.

Heat the remaining oil in the skillet over medium-high heat and add the remaining ginger and garlic, the carrots, bell pepper, snow peas and scallions. Cook, stirring, for 2 to 3 minutes, or until the vegetables just begin to lose their bright color. Stir the stock mixture to recombine it, then add it to the skillet. Add the shrimp mixture and the red pepper flakes, and bring the mixture to a boil, stirring constantly. Boil the mixture for 2 to 3 minutes, or until the sauce thickens and the shrimp are firm. Divide the rice among 4 plates, top with the shrimp mixture and serve. Makes 4 servings

CALORIES per serving	381
55% Carbohydrate	52 g
15% Protein	14 g
30% Fat	13 g
CALCIUM	80 mg
IRON	4 mg
SODIUM	343 mg

SPANAKOPITA

Cottage cheese and yogurt — in the form of creamy yogurt cheese — supply most of the calcium in this Greek cheese-and-spinach pie.

2 cups plain lowfat yogurt	1 tablespoon chopped fresh dill,
1 pound spinach	or 1 teaspoon dried dill
3/4 cup lowfat cottage	2 teaspoons grated lemon peel
cheese (1%)	1/2 teaspoon white pepper
3 tablespoons unbleached	1/4 teaspoon salt
all-purpose flour	3 tablespoons margarine
1 cup chopped scallions	8 sheets phyllo dough
1/4 cup chopped fresh parsley	

To make the yogurt cheese, place a cheesecloth-lined strainer over a bowl. Spoon the yogurt into the strainer, cover with plastic wrap and refrigerate for 24 hours, or until the yogurt is the consistency of thick sour cream. You should have about 1

CALORIES per serving	375
52% Carbohydrate	50 g
21% Protein	20 g
27% Fat	11 g
CALCIUM	350 mg
IRON	5 mg
SODIUM	555 mg

cup of yogurt cheese. (Discard the whey, or reserve it to use in soups or in baking recipes requiring buttermilk or sour milk.)

Trim and wash thoroughly but do not dry the spinach. Place it in a large saucepan over medium-high heat, cover and cook, stirring 2 or 3 times, for 1 to 2 minutes, or until the spinach is limp. Drain it in a colander, pressing out as much of the water as possible, then set the spinach aside to drain and cool completely.

Preheat the oven to 375° F. In a large bowl stir together the yogurt cheese, cottage cheese, flour, scallions, parsley, dill, lemon peel, pepper and salt. Squeeze any excess moisture from the spinach. Coarsely chop the spinach and add it to the cheese mixture; set aside. Melt the margarine in a small saucepan over medium-low heat; set aside.

Unfold the phyllo and cover it with a damp kitchen towel (keep the phyllo covered while you work to keep it from drying out). Place 1 sheet of phyllo in a 9-inch tart pan (preferably with a removable bottom), and brush it lightly with margarine. Place another sheet of phyllo in the pan at right angles to the first to form a cross, and brush it with margarine. Layer in the remaining phyllo sheets in crisscross fashion to form an even overhang of pastry around the pan, brushing each sheet with margarine. Spoon the cheese mixture into the pan and fold the phyllo over it to cover it completely. Brush the top with the remaining margarine and bake the spanakopita for 15 to 20 minutes, or until golden brown. Carefully remove the sides of the pan, leaving the spanakopita on the pan bottom, and transfer it to a platter. (If using a regular tart pan, serve directly from the pan.) Cut the spanakopita into quarters and serve.

Makes 4 servings

ONION SOUP WITH SHALLOT TOASTS

Unlike traditional French onion soup, this is a purée with thin, crisp cheese toasts on top. The leeks supply most of the calcium in this dish.

2 cups low-sodium chicken stock	1 bay leaf
4 cups coarsely chopped leeks	1/8 teaspoon white pepper
1 cup coarsely chopped onion	1 tablespoon margarine
2 garlic cloves, chopped	1 cup coarsely chopped shallots
2 tablespoons sherry	6 ounces Italian bread
1/2 teaspoon dried thyme	2 tablespoons grated Parmesan

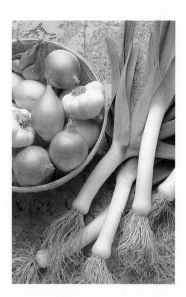

In a medium-size saucepan combine the stock, leeks, onion, garlic, sherry, thyme, bay leaf, white pepper and 1 1/2 cups of water, and bring to a boil over medium-high heat. Cover, reduce the heat to low and simmer for 1 hour.

Remove and discard the bay leaf. Using a slotted spoon, transfer the solids from the soup to a food processor or blender and process until puréed. Return the purée to the pan, cover and set aside.

Preheat the broiler. Meanwhile, melt the margarine in a small skillet over medium-high heat, add the shallots and sauté for 1 to 2 minutes, or until they begin to brown. Toast the bread slices under the broiler for 1 minute on each side, or until golden; set aside. Reheat the soup over medium-high heat, stirring occasionally, for 3 to 5 minutes, or until heated through. Meanwhile, divide the shallots among the slices of toast, sprinkle them with Parmesan and broil for another minute, or until golden brown and fragrant. Divide the soup among 4 bowls, top with toast and serve. *Makes 4 servings*

CALORIES per serving	283
71% Carbohydrate	51 g
13% Protein	9 g
16% Fat	5 g
CALCIUM	138 mg
IRON	5 mg
SODIUM	383 mg

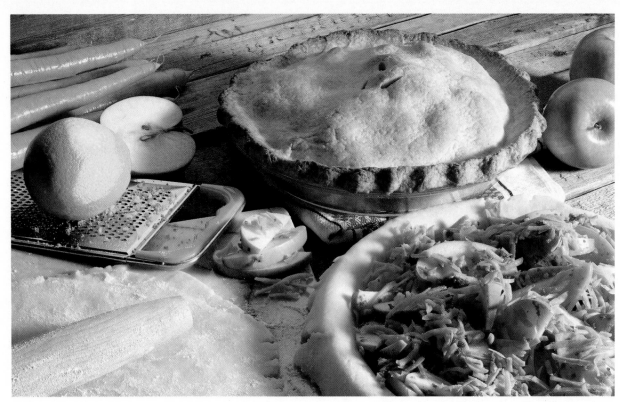

Apple-Carrot Pie

Desserts

APPLE-CARROT PIE

The carrots and apples each contribute about 70 milligrams of potassium to a serving of this pie.

CALORIES per serving	249
66% Carbohydrate	42 g
5% Protein	3 g
29% Fat	9 g
CALCIUM	30mg
IRON	1 mg
SODIUM	137 mg

1 1/2 cups plus 2 tablespoons
   unbleached all-purpose flour
2 tablespoons granulated sugar
Pinch of salt
7 tablespoons margarine
3 Granny Smith apples (about
   1 1/2 pounds total weight)
2 cups grated carrots

1/2 cup fresh bread crumbs,
   preferably pumpernickel
1/2 cup brown sugar
2 tablespoons orange juice
1 tablespoon grated orange peel
1 tablespoon grated fresh ginger
1/2 teaspoon ground cinnamon

In a medium-size bowl stir together 1 1/2 cups of flour, the granulated sugar and salt. Using a pastry blender or 2 knives, cut the margarine into the dry ingredients until the mixture resembles coarse cornmeal. Add 3 to 4 tablespoons of cold water and stir until the dough forms a cohesive mass. Knead the dough for 1 minute, then form it into a ball, flatten it into a disk and wrap it in plastic wrap. Refrigerate the dough for 20 minutes. Meanwhile, wash and core but do not peel the apples, and cut them into 1/4-inch-thick wedges. Place the apples in a large bowl and add the carrots, bread crumbs, brown sugar, orange juice and peel, ginger and cinnamon. Toss the mixture to coat the apples and carrots with orange juice and set aside.

Preheat the oven 425° F. Lightly flour the work surface and rolling pin. Set aside one third of the dough. Roll out the remaining dough to an 12-inch disk and carefully transfer it to a 9-inch pie pan. Press the dough into the pan, then fill it with the apple mixture, packing the filling down lightly. Dust the work surface and rolling pin with flour again. Roll out the remaining dough to a 9-inch circle, place it on the filling and crimp together the edges of the bottom and top crusts. Make two or three 1/2-inch slashes in the top crust with a sharp knife. Bake the pie for 15 minutes, then reduce the oven temperature to 350° F. and bake for 15 to 20 minutes more, or until the crust is golden brown. Let the pie cool on a rack for 10 minutes and serve it warm, or cool it completely and serve it at room temperature.

Makes 10 servings

SWEET POTATO-BANANA PUDDING

No sugar is necessary when sweet potatoes and bananas are combined. The potatoes are an outstanding source of vitamin A.

CALORIES per serving		249
76% Carbohydrate		50 g
5% Protein		3 g
19% Fat		6 g
CALCIUM		29 mg
IRON		1 mg
SODIUM		13 mg

1 pound cooked, cooled
  sweet potatoes
4 bananas

1/2 teaspoon ground nutmeg
1/2 teaspoon vanilla extract
1 ounce chopped pecans

Peel and mash the sweet potatoes; set aside. Peel the bananas and purée them in a food processor or blender, then add the mashed potatoes, nutmeg and vanilla, and process for 5 to 10 seconds, or until blended. Divide the pudding among 4 dessert dishes, sprinkle with pecans and serve. The pudding can also be refrigerated for 2 to 3 hours and served chilled.   Makes 4 servings

FLAMBEED BANANAS AND APPLES

Bananas and pistachio nuts are excellent sources of potassium and magnesium; the pistachios are used only as a garnish because they are high in fat.

2 tablespoons unsweetened
  frozen apple juice concentrate
Pinch of ground nutmeg
1 banana

1 apple
1 1/2 teaspoons margarine
1 tablespoon rum
2 teaspoons chopped pistachios

Stir together the apple juice concentrate and nutmeg in a cup; set aside. Peel the banana and cut it into 1/2-inch diagonal slices. Core the apple and slice it into 1/4-inch-thick wedges. Melt the margarine in a medium-size nonstick skillet over medium-high heat. Add the apples and cook, turning the slices to cook them evenly, for 1 minute, or until they just begin to brown. Add the banana slices, and cook, turning them to coat them with margarine, for 30 to 60 seconds, or until they just begin to soften. Add the apple juice mixture, bring to a boil and cook for 1 minute; set aside. In a small skillet, heat the rum over low heat for 10 to 15 seconds. Carefully ignite the rum with a match and pour the burning rum over the fruit. When the flame goes out, divide the fruit and sauce between 2 plates and top with pistachios.   Makes 2 servings

CALORIES per serving		180
73% Carbohydrate		32 g
3% Protein		1 g
24% Fat		5 g
CALCIUM		17 mg
IRON		1 mg
SODIUM		39 mg

Snacks and Beverages

POTATO ROLLS

You can make these rolls with either white or sweet potato. Sweet potatoes contain four times the calcium of white potatoes, but white potatoes have much more potassium.

CALORIES per roll made with white potatoes	247
78% Carbohydrate	48 g
10% Protein	6 g
12% Fat	3 g
CALCIUM	53 mg
IRON	2 mg
SODIUM	50 mg

1/4 pound white or sweet potato
1 cup buttermilk
1 cup dark raisins
2 tablespoons vegetable oil
2 tablespoons sugar

1 package dry yeast
3 1/4 cups unbleached
   all-purpose flour, approximately
2 tablespoons nonfat dry milk
Pinch of salt

Place the potato in a small saucepan with cold water to cover it, and bring to a boil over medium-high heat. Cover the pan, reduce the heat to medium-low, and cook the potato for 20 minutes, or until tender when pierced with a knife. When the potato is cooked, set it aside to cool slightly; reserve the cooking water.

Potato Rolls

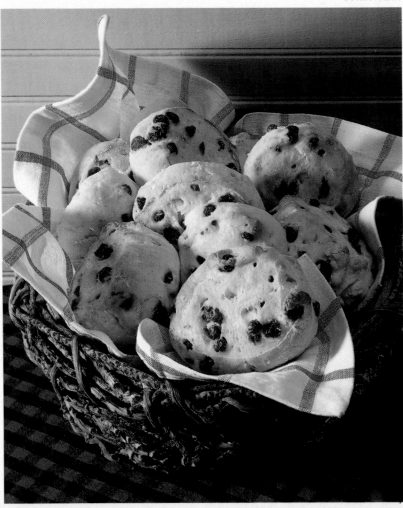

Peel the potato, mash it in a small bowl, then stir in the buttermilk, raisins and oil; set aside. In a small bowl combine 1/4 cup of the warm cooking water and 1 tablespoon of sugar. Add the yeast and let the mixture stand for 1 to 2 minutes, or until the yeast begins to foam. Meanwhile, combine 3 1/4 cups of flour, the dry milk, 1 tablespoon of sugar and the salt in a medium-size bowl and make a well in the center. Pour in the potato and yeast mixtures and stir until well combined. Turn the dough onto a lightly floured surface and knead it for 5 to 7 minutes, or until smooth, dusting it with more flour if necessary to prevent sticking. Place the dough in a clean medium-size bowl, cover it with a kitchen towel and set aside in a warm place to rise for 40 minutes, or until doubled in bulk.

Punch down the dough and knead it on a floured surface for 1 minute. Roll it into a 20-inch-long rope about 2 inches thick, cut the rope into ten 2-inch sections and place them on a baking sheet. Set aside to rise for 25 minutes.

Preheat the oven to 350° F. Bake the rolls for 15 to 20 minutes, or until golden brown on top. Let cool slightly before serving. Makes 10 servings

SPICY SQUASH SHAKE

Calcium and phosphorus, found in the milk, tofu and squash, make this lowfat shake nutritious as well as refreshing.

1/2 cup cooked butternut squash, well chilled	1/2 cup skim milk
1 ounce tofu (2 tablespoons)	Pinch of ground ginger
1 tablespoon honey	Pinch of pumpkin pie spice

Combine the squash, tofu and honey in a blender and process for 10 seconds, or until smooth. Add the milk and spices, and process for another 5 seconds. Pour the shake into a glass and serve. Makes 1 serving

CALORIES per serving	170
76% Carbohydrate	35 g
16% Protein	7 g
8% Fat	2 g
CALCIUM	224 mg
IRON	2 mg
SODIUM	71 mg

BANANA-BERRY GELATIN

A banana-berry gelatin dessert mix, consisting mostly of sugar and artificial flavoring, has 90 milligrams of sodium per serving. Using naturally sweet grape juice and fresh fruit, you need much less sugar to make this dessert, which contains minimal sodium and about 500 milligrams of potassium per serving.

1 envelope unflavored gelatin	1/2 cup fresh or frozen raspberries
1 tablespoon lemon juice	r 2 tablespoons sugar
4 bananas, peeled and mashed	2 tablespoons toasted wheat germ
1 cup unsweetened grape juice	

Stir together the gelatin, lemon juice and 1/2 cup of warm water in a small saucepan. Allow the gelatin to soften for 30 seconds, then stir the mixture gently over medium-low heat until the gelatin dissolves completely. Remove the pan from the heat, add the bananas, grape juice, raspberries and sugar, and stir until well blended. Divide the mixture among 4 dessert dishes and refrigerate for 2 to 3 hours, or until the gelatin is firm. Just before serving, sprinkle the desserts with wheat germ. Makes 4 servings

CALORIES per serving	197
89% Carbohydrate	47 g
7% Protein	4 g
4% Fat	1 g
CALCIUM	19 mg
IRON	1 mg
SODIUM	4 mg

PROP CREDITS

Cover: tank top–Athletic Style, New York City, shorts–Hind Performance Sportswear, San Luis Obispo, Calif., sneakers–Avia, Alexandria, Va.; page 7: tank top and tights–Athletic Style, New York City, sneakers–Nautilus Athletic Footwear, Inc., Greenville, S.C.; pages 26-43: tights–Hind Performance Sportswear, San Luis Obispo, Calif.; pages 44-55: leotard–Marika, courtesy of The Weekend Exercise Co., San Diego, Calif., tights–Hind Performance Sportswear, San Luis Obispo, Calif.; pages 56-57: tank top–Hind Performance Sportswear, San Luis Obispo, Calif.; pages 60-61: tank top and shorts–Hind Performance Sportswear, San Luis Obispo, Calif.; pages 60-91: mats courtesy of Jodi's Gym, New York City; pages 62-65: leotard and tights–Dance France, LTD, Santa Monica, Calif.; pages 66-71: tank top and shorts–Hind Performance Sportswear, San Luis Obispo, Calif.; pages 72-79: leotard and tights–Dance France, LTD, Santa Monica, Calif.; pages 80-83: tank top and shorts–Hind Performance Sportswear, San Luis Obispo, Calif., sneakers–Avia, Alexandria, Va.; pages 84-87: leotard and tights–Dance France, LTD, Santa Monica, Calif., shorts–Hind Performance Sportswear, San Luis Obispo, Calif., sneakers–Avia, Alexandria, Va.; pages 88-91: tank top and shorts–Hind Performance Sportswear, San Luis Obispo, Calif.; pages 92-93: gray tights–Super Runners Shop, New York City; pages 96-123: leotards and tights–Dance France, LTD, Santa Monica, Calif., tank tops and shorts–Athletic Style, New York City; page 128: tiles–Country Floors, New York City, napkin–Frank MacIntosh at Henri Bendel, New York City; page 131: plates–Gear Stores, New York City; page 134: plates–Sweet Nellie, New York City, salad servers and napkin–Frank MacIntosh at Henri Bendel, New York City, salad-dressing pitcher–Simon Pearce, New York City.

ACKNOWLEDGMENTS

All cosmetics and grooming products supplied by Clinique Labs, Inc., New York City

Nutrition analysis provided by Hill Nutrition Associates, Fayetteville, N.Y.

Off-camera warm-up equipment: rowing machine supplied by Precor USA, Redmond, Wash.; Tunturi stationary bicycle supplied by Amerec Corp., Bellevue, Wash.

Washing machine and dryer supplied by White-Westinghouse, Columbus, Ohio

Index prepared by Ian Tucker

Production by Giga Communications

PHOTOGRAPHY CREDITS

Exercise photographs by Andrew Eccles; food photographs by Steven Mays, Rebus, Inc.

ILLUSTRATION CREDITS

Pages 8-9, 11, 14, 21, illustrations: David Flaherty; pages 18-19, 59, illustrations: Kevin Kelly.

Time-Life Books Inc. offers a wide range of fine recordings, including a Rock 'n' Roll Era *series. For subscription information, call 1-800-621-7026, or write TIME-LIFE MUSIC, P. O. Box C-32068; Richmond, Virginia 23261-2068.*

INDEX

One-knee roll, 66, 68-69
osteoporosis, 127

Partner exercises, 17, 93-123
  balance, 94-95
  spotting, 95
  strength-building, 94, 100-105
  stretching, 96-99
periodontal disease, 127
phosphorus, 125, 126
pike jump, 87
plateaus in training, 16
plié, 25
potassium, 125-127
practice, 12-13, 15
proprioception, 10-11, 57
protein
  amounts in recipe dishes, 128-141
  recommended intake of, 127
push-ups, 32-33, 102-103

Recipes
  beverage, 141
  breakfast, 128-130
  dessert, 138-139
  dinner, 134-137
  lunch, 131-133

snack, 140-141
relevé, 25
rolls
  backward, 72-79
  forward, 58, 66-71
roundoffs, 86, 90-91

Safety, 17, 20
scale, 25
self-assessment, 16-19
shoes, for tumbling, 58
shoulder stand, 73
sit-up, negative, test, 17, 18
snack recipes, 140-141
sodium, 125
  amounts in recipe dishes, 128-141
  restriction of intake, 126, 127
somersault, 25
spotters, 17, 20, 25, 57, 80, 95
squats, 100-101
straddle roll
  backward, 78-79
  forward, 66, 68-69
straight jump, 86
strength-building exercises, 26-35, 94,
  100-105
stretching
  at the barre, 36-43

on the floor, 26-35
importance of, 16
partner, 96-99

Transverse axis, 59
tripod balance, 81
tuck jump, 86
tumbling, 57-91
  backward rolls, 72-79
  balancing, 58, 80-85
  body strength and, 58
  cartwheels, 86, 88-89
  clothes for, 58
  conditioners, 60-65
  exercise mats for, 58
  forward rolls, 58, 66-71
  jumps, 86-87
  performance in other sports
    and, 17
  proprioception and, 57
  roundoffs, 86, 90-91
  safety and, 20
  space for, 58
  three axes of movement, 59
turnout, 25

Warming up, 24